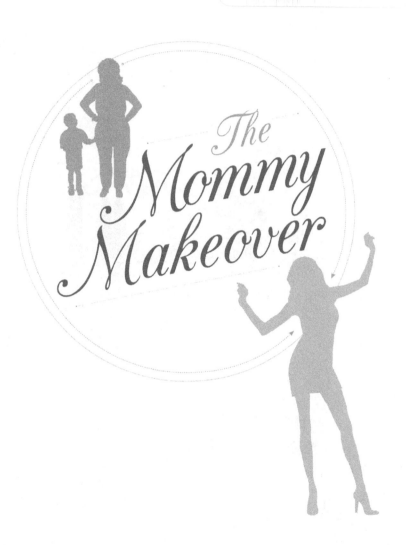

The Mommy Makeover

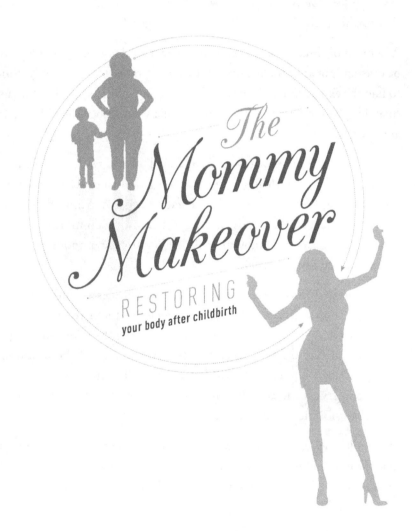

The Mommy Makeover

RESTORING
your body after childbirth

MICHAEL R. BURGDORF, MD, MPH

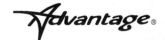

More praise for *The Mommy Makeover*

"Hooray for *The Mommy Makeover!* I am so thankful that Dr. Mike is sharing the truth about the gift of plastic surgery!

As a mom of three sons, a busy entrepreneur, and a woman determined to be outstanding at both, 'me time' is extremely rare! It was not only difficult to find the extra time in the day to devote to my needs, it was hard to justify spending the money on myself—there are always things the children need and everyday life expenses.

Thankfully, with encouragement from David, my fantastic friend and hair-dresser, and from Dr. Mike, I began making time and placing priority on how I look and feel about myself… I started my own Mommy Makeover! What a difference it has made in my life! I am so much more confident in how I look and what I can wear. It is thrilling to be a grandmother and be complimented about my 'look!' Why did I wait so long?

The Mommy Makeover explains the procedures clearly and outlines the vast opportunities available to help you feel good about yourself again. Dr. Mike has a gift, and he knows the obstacles women face (real or imagined) when considering plastic surgery. If you've ever wondered about how to get your pre-baby body back, Dr. Mike covers it all—from deciding to have plastic surgery to choosing the right doctor, even dealing with your home and responsibilities during recovery.

This book is a great reminder to me and other women that it's so important to care for myself in order to invest in others (my family, my employees, my community). It's time for your Mommy Makeover—see what a difference it can make!"

—Cordia Harrington,
also known as "The BunLady", is founder and CEO of The Bun Companies, a $100mm bakery enterprise serving the most elite customers in the US and Caribbean. She is also a community volunteer and serves on the boards of publicly-owned companies.

"As a former patient of Dr. Burgdorf, I can honestly say that *The Mommy Makeover* is a completely accurate reflection of him as a doctor and person. When searching for a plastic surgeon, it was extremely important to me to find a skilled doctor I can trust. It also was very important to find a doctor that will take time to listen, care, and address my concerns and questions. Dr. Burgdorf did all of that. I was extremely impressed with him after our first consult. I knew I had found an exceptional doctor. From start to finish, I have been extremely pleased with my results! I just can't say enough about Dr. Burgdorf. He has made my dreams come true. It was one of the best decisions I ever made trusting him with my Mommy Makeover, honestly!

For any mom even just thinking about making a change to her body, *The Mommy Makeover* is a must read. I was lucky enough to get this information in person, but reading this book was like being in the consultation all over again. He outlines and addresses all the fears and concerns a mom might experience and offers solutions to overcome them. He has thought of everything involved with these procedures.

I loved this book because it reminded me of my own journey to regain my body. If you are considering a Mommy Makeover, stop what you are doing, put the kids to bed, get them a play date, do whatever you can to find time to read The Mommy Makeover before going any further! You'll be happy you did, I promise."

—**Mandy McDaniel**
Mother

"As a busy working mom of two young kids, time is not something I have a whole lot of. Dr. Mike's book has provided me with invaluable information—all in one place—about my options when it comes to taking care of myself and my body. This book is a fantastic resource for understanding exactly what goes into the Mommy Makeover and addresses all of the questions that I could possibly think of. It takes the guessing game out of it completely and also takes away some of the fear surrounding the procedures. Because Dr. Mike is also a husband and dad, I know that he has looked at this topic from more than just a surgeon's perspective and that is important to me as a wife and mom. I can't wait to pass this along to my mommy friends!"

—**Suzi Ellis**
luxury brand publicist and small business owner

"As an OB/GYN, I understand the intimate doctor/patient relationship, the unique emotions a mother experiences, and have seen, first hand, the effects of childbirth on a mom. In *The Mommy Makeover*, Dr. Mike Burgdorf expertly manages this relationship, handles these emotions, and skillfully guides a mom through the process of deciding upon and continuing through with plastic surgery to restore her body.

This book offers a tiny glimpse of the sensitivity he displays when dealing with his patients. Dr. Mike Burgdorf is a gifted surgeon, a master communicator, and a respected member of our community, as well as a good friend. I trust him with my patients and my family and can't wait to share this book with them."

—Christopher M. Sizemore, DO, FACOG
Assistant Professor
Obstetrics and Gynecology
Vanderbilt Center for Women's Health

Published by Advantage, Charleston, South Carolina.
Member of Advantage Media Group.

ADVANTAGE is a registered trademark and the Advantage colophon is a trademark of Advantage Media Group, Inc.

Printed in the United States of America.

ISBN: 978-1-59932-517-0
LCCN: 2015943497

This publication is designed to provide accurate and authoritative information in regard to the subject matter covered. It is sold with the understanding that the publisher is not engaged in rendering legal, accounting, or other professional services. If legal advice or other expert assistance is required, the services of a competent professional person should be sought.

This book is not meant to diagnose, treat, or offer specific individual medical advice and should not be used in place of seeking qualified medical care. By reading this book, the reader agrees to hold harmless the publisher, author, and/or all associated entities from acts or omissions taken as a result of information or opinions expressed in this book.

Advantage Media Group is proud to be a part of the Tree Neutral® program. Tree Neutral offsets the number of trees consumed in the production and printing of this book by taking proactive steps such as planting trees in direct proportion to the number of trees used to print books. To learn more about Tree Neutral, please visit www.treeneutral.com. To learn more about Advantage's commitment to being a responsible steward of the environment, please visit www.advantagefamily.com/green

Advantage Media Group is a publisher of business, self-improvement, and professional development books and online learning. We help entrepreneurs, business leaders, and professionals share their Stories, Passion, and Knowledge to help others Learn & Grow. Do you have a manuscript or book idea that you would like us to consider for publishing? Please visit advantagefamily.com or call 1.866.775.1696.

To my Mom,
who set the standard on being a Mom. Her love for her children is
immeasurable, her sacrifices too numerous to count, and her dedication
to her family is unsurpassed. I am so lucky to have you for a mom.

To Casey,
in raising four children and working as a physician, you have brought
a new meaning to the label "Mom". You have helped mold our legacy
and, in turn, have helped me become the man I'm meant to be.

ACKNOWLEDGEMENTS

To all of my patients, I am truly indebted to you for trusting me with your time, your life, and your beauty. Thank you for allowing me to perform my "dream job" in helping you achieve your desired transformation.

I also owe special thanks to Connie "Hacksaw" LeBeau whose tireless effort to edit this manuscript has been invaluable.

TABLE OF CONTENTS

My Path to Plastic Surgery

When writing this book, I took careful consideration to make sure my voice and my personality came through accurately. Not because this book is about me but because you'll be listening to me a lot throughout our time together. This book is about mothers and their individual struggles with considering and undergoing a major change in their body image. I want you to get to know me in a real way, not just by reading the accomplishments, awards, and degrees from the back cover or my website. I want to show you who I am and why I care in an informative, comforting, encouraging, and helpful manner as we navigate together, starting with this book, the wonderful world of reclaiming your body—and your sense of your self—through the Mommy Makeover.

My name is Michael R. Burgdorf, MD, MPH, usually just known as Dr. Mike. I grew up in New Jersey as part of a large, and forever-expanding, blended family. My parents divorced when I was quite young and each subsequently remarried. What started out as a traditional family of four turned into an exciting and chaotic arena of stepbrothers, stepsisters, and half sisters from both sides of the family tree. With a total of six siblings on one side and five on the other, and many of us now married with children of our own, you can imagine the circus we affectionately call family holidays.

I had the benefit of growing up with two strong and loving male role models, my father and my stepfather, both very successful and accomplished businessmen. But my mother was the constant and guiding presence in my life. She cheered me on daily. She sacrificed a significant portion of her day to get me to a school near my father's house so I could get a good education and maintain a relationship with him. She taught me to dance. She taught me how to relate to and communicate with girls. She taught me how to be sensitive to others, how to be tough when I was sad, and the importance of being kind even when I felt angry. As a registered nurse, she inspired my interest in the medical world by recounting tales of her experiences working in the operating room. My mom is special to me; we share a bond like no other in my life.

Thankfully, my mom is not the squeamish type, and she allowed me to start playing football in the fourth grade. She encouraged me in this sport from the beginning, not realizing the huge impact it would have on my life. I played throughout high school and am proud to have played linebacker for the University of Notre Dame under the legendary coach Lou Holtz. Coach Holtz's commitment to excellence in all parts of life was exemplified by his WIN (What's Important Now?) philosophy. While embracing this philosophy as a young student athlete, I played football and maintained a sharp focus on academics, which got me invited to the academic excellence banquet each year at Notre Dame and, ultimately, earned my admission to medical school. And I still ask myself that WIN question on a regular basis.

Lou Holtz would often say, "People don't care how much you know until they know how much you care." That belief truly changed my life. At the end of practice or after a game, coach would often say something like, "All right, men, it's important to realize that the words we speak and the actions we take can affect people in a very profound way. Always consider the sensitivities and the needs of those around you. Be aware of how your actions hinder or help someone." I strive every day to live this lesson in my medical practice and my life in general. "Consider the sensitivities"—while that may seem unusual coming from the football world, it has become my mantra in many aspects of my life.

So has "Do the right thing." Coach punctuated our Friday night practices with a relaxation session during which he would talk to us about being honest with ourselves. "Men, you can fool the television cameras, the fans, even your friends and family ... but not yourself. At the end of the day, you have to look at yourself in the mirror and know that what you did was the right thing to do." I hold this philosophy dear in my life, want it to always be a part of my character, and teach it to my own children. I want to live my life openly and honestly with the highest of integrity à la Lou Holtz, imparting the skills I have developed—intellectually, personally, professionally—with kindness and compassion.

Thanks, Coach, for all this and for so much more.

I moved from the gridiron to the Big Easy when I finished undergrad and attended medical school at Tulane University in New Orleans. The day I was accepted to Tulane, my top-choice school, I was playing in the Notre Dame versus Navy game in Ireland: truly one of my lifetime's top-ten moments.

Ah, New Orleans! I loved being there for medical school and other obvious reasons—the people, the food, the music, and riding on some floats in Mardi Gras. I was also there to study—and study I did! During my first year in medical school, an opportunity arose to earn my masters in public health (MPH) concurrent with my doctorate in medicine (MD). I jumped at the chance. I also trained at the renowned Charity Hospital. I wanted to have a tough, demanding medical education, and that's exactly what I got. Day one of medical school: I show up at Charity's emergency room. A doctor I had never seen before called to me, "Hey you! Here! [Hands me a chart.] Go sew up bed four!" It was sink or swim, and my first lesson, loud and clear, was "If you show up, Dr. Mike, you better be prepared." I decided I was never going to "practice" on people, never going to think in terms of bed numbers, never going to see a patient as a disease instead of a human being. In my clinic today, there are no numbers on the room doors; we call our patients by their names, not their condition being treated.

I stayed in New Orleans at Tulane for my surgical residency. My world there was filled with chaos and trauma, a battlefield of real, raw, bare—and very human—need. And here, in the midst of all this, was a young surgeon's opportunity to bring calm, quiet confidence, compassion, and efficiency to an environment that was anything but controlled. One night, very early in my tenure there, three gunshot victims rolled in in rapid succession. I was in Room One, when the attending surgeon steps in, grabs my hand, and guides it to the patient's chest and says, "Open him up stem to stern." The room was suddenly filled with blood and guts—and tension. This guy's life was literally in our hands. The attending remained calm and cool, spoke quietly and directly, moved quickly, and helped me stop the hemorrhaging. "If you're the captain of the ship and you behave as if it's sinking," he told me later over coffee, "everyone around you will panic. If you remain calm and decisive, even if you are standing in knee-deep water, the sailors will grab some pails and start bailing. You did that earlier. Thanks for captaining the ship with me tonight."

And on the subject of deep water ... My residency at Tulane ended prematurely and abruptly when Hurricane Katrina hit New Orleans. I left in a rush on Sunday, the day Katrina made landfall in New Orleans, to ensure the safety of my wife, my only son at the time, and our family dog. It was my plan to get them to Mississippi, leave them in the charge of my in-laws, and return quickly. That was not to be because of the timing of the storm and the disastrous flooding that ensued. While the work I did in a makeshift clinic in Jackson, Mississippi, at the time was still important, for a guy who had spent many months preparing professionally and emotionally for such events, this was but a poor substitute for what I felt and, in some ways still feel, was what I was *really* meant to be doing in New Orleans that week. It still tears at me today.

I have had to draw on my strong faith, belief in God, and an understanding that I am where I am, doing what I am supposed to do, for good reasons that I may not yet comprehend. Just as I learned to be calm and efficient in the face of the world called Charity Hospital, I have had to learn how to face the chaos, the trauma, the lack of control that was Katrina and the circumstances that prevented me from being there to help. I continue to draw on the resiliency, the belief, the faith that I am meant to bring goodness to the lives of many and that God will guide me in doing it well, for the right reasons, each and every day.

Because my wife's family was in Mississippi, we chose to stay there after Katrina. I had already determined that plastic surgery was my passion. After finishing my general surgery residency, I was blessed to be able to complete my plastic surgery residency at the University of Mississippi in Jackson, home to one of the largest plastic surgery groups in the US.

And speaking of Mississippi, I would be remiss if I didn't mention my wife when trying to provide insight into myself. My wife has been my perfect partner through life. She has provided me with a beautiful family and, as a physician herself, understands the crazy life of a doctor as only one who lives it can. As any working mom does, she struggles daily with the pull of her career (her patients adore her) and her family. But she's really good at both. I mean *really* good. Even though she has put aside her goals and desires to allow me to pursue my own, has sacrificed her body and her sanity to become pregnant four times, and helps raise our four children, she still keeps it all together. She keeps all that medical knowledge at the front of her brain (even during her "baby brain" phase of pregnancy). She's forever gentle and loving to our kids and worries about the tiniest detail in their lives. I don't know how she does it … she just takes care of things. She is the best woman I know, in all senses, is the best mother to our children that I could ever ask for, and has ceaselessly supported me in my life, as well as my career as a plastic surgeon.

I love the creative and artistic parts of plastic surgery as much as I love the technical challenges. I love restoring self-confidence in my patients, improving their lives, and helping them see themselves in a renewed light. Plastic surgery allows me to have a significant impact on many peoples' lives. What's exciting for me is that the impact seems to extend like a ripple in the water. I help make changes on the outside of an individual. Then I can be a witness to the countless changes that occur on the inside of that same person. The effects on people within that person's sphere can be profound. With Mommy Makeovers, that ripple effect can permeate through an entire family. To me, that is just so special.

The specific procedures for a Mommy Makeover are important, as are the skills of the individual surgeon. I am aware, however, that my ability to make these changes in someone else is not solely dependent upon my skill alone or the procedures chosen. I depend on God for the skills I have and the opportunities I receive. Before each surgery, I ask him to guide me and my hands and allow me to achieve the results I am trying to obtain and which the patient desires.

I bring my knowledge; skills and experience; integrity and character; commitment to excellence; a kind, caring, compassionate heart; and a strong faith to the world of my practice and my patients in Nashville. I try to be someone who maintains perspective that the patients' desires, concerns, and fears are very real. I try to be a person who treats others like I would like to be treated.

I hope that offers some insight into Dr. Mike Burgdorf and allows you to trust me as we go through this joyful journey of rejuvenation in exploring the Mommy Makeover together. Thanks for taking the first step with me.

MOMMY MAKEOVER MYTHS

Myth: Exercise can lift and augment your breasts naturally.

Reality: Not so. You can exercise hours every day, and your breasts will still be droopy. Your pectoral muscles will be in good shape, but the size of your breasts won't change.

Myth: You can't breast-feed after a breast lift.

Reality: While this hasn't been completely proven one way or the other, the consensus is that about two-thirds of all women can breast-feed before breast surgery; about two-thirds can breast-feed afterward. It is important to choose an experienced, board-certified plastic surgeon who knows how to preserve breast function.

Myth: If you have breast implants, a mammogram can rupture them.

Reality: Unlikely to occur, unless there are capsular contractures present (see chapter 16).

Myth: Exercise will tighten your tummy and get you back to the way you were before the baby.

Reality: No amount of exercise can tighten up fibrous tissue that has been stretched by pregnancy.

Myth: Rubbing creams into your abdomen and breasts will prevent stretch marks.

Reality: When the skin is stretched by the natural swelling of pregnancy and breast-feeding, the marks may fade a bit, but they are permanent, a form of scarring. The best practice is to reduce the problem by maintaining good hydration and having moderate weight gain throughout pregnancy.

Myth: If you have liposuction, you can't regain weight in that area.
Reality: Yes, you can. With large weight gain, you can actually eat through the liposuction.

Myth: A Mommy Makeover isn't safe.
Reality: All surgery has some risk, but a Mommy Makeover is very safe when performed by an experienced, board-certified plastic surgeon.

Myth: You will look plastic or fake after the surgery.
Reality: A skilled surgeon will give you natural-looking results. Subtlety is key.

Myth: Everybody will know I had surgery.
Reality: Only if you tell them—which I hope you do and refer them to me as patients.

Myth: My husband just won't understand.
Reality: You don't know that until you talk about it. He may surprise you and be very supportive—that has been my experience with my patients over the years.

Myth: I can't afford it.
Reality: Yes, a Mommy Makeover costs real money and is not covered by insurance. Think of it as an investment in yourself.

Myth: I'm not worth it.
Reality: Yes, you are.

Myth: I'm not ready to have such confidence.
Reality: Look out, world!

Myth: I'll never get my body back to what it was before my baby.
Reality: Oh, yes you will! Your Mommy Makeover will amaze you.

Part 1

DECISIONS

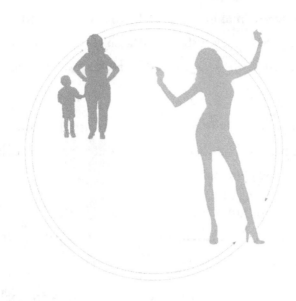

Chapter 1

MOM, ISN'T IT TIME FOR *YOU*?

5:30 a.m.: Baby is stirring … Ugh! Gotta get out of bed … Hurry! Get the bottle ready, and get her changed so she doesn't wake the rest of the house. Oops, too late. Here come the boys …

6:00 a.m.: Okay, time for breakfast … Cereal for one, eggs for another, third one not hungry this morning. "How about a cereal bar, honey?"

6:30 a.m.: Noise, chaos, so much noise … and the endless moving parts of backpacks, lunch boxes, plates, cups, and silverware. "Come on, finish eating so you don't miss the bus." Jackets on, shoes on …

head on a swivel, making sure each one is accounted for with the appropriate garb as they rush out to catch the bus. "Don't forget your lunch. Good luck on your test today. Here's your jacket. Wait! Your backpack!"

7:45 a.m.: Whew! Why am I so exhausted before 8:00 a.m.? Maybe the baby will go back to sleep, and I can nap with her for a bit. I'll go to the gym tomorrow.

8:10 a.m.: Guilt overriding any thoughts of sleep. I need to do the laundry, clean up the kitchen, and organize that pantry. Breakfast for me? Later. Makeup? In the car …

And you pick the scenario: I've got to get to work, baby's crying again, etc.

The day goes on at this hectic pace and only mildly slows when the kids are at school.

You start each day hopeful and think you'll be fine. Most times your thoughts revolve around your kids. You worry. Are you teaching them well, are they making the right friends, fitting in, have we signed up for the right activities, will they grow up to be kind, thoughtful, empathetic, etc.? You make it through the day, barely, and still don't exercise or even get a short nap.

Afterschool activities ramp up the harried schedule again, and you are living in the car. But you're good. You're organized. You're Mom. After going through your checklist of diaper bag, diapers, wipes, baby food, coloring books, homework, etc., you realize you forgot your phone. Again. Oh well, you're needed to help with homework anyway; they'll leave a message if it's important.

The schedule basically repeats itself in reverse for the nighttime activities. Sit down for dinner? Yeah, right! Unless it's done in your car. For your meal, it's either fast food to accommodate the kids, or it's stealing bites of mac 'n' cheese from your child's plate as you race around the kitchen to make sure everyone else is fed and satisfied. And you are exhausted. Will you ever find time for yourself?

It's rare for a mom to think of herself first—they usually put themselves last, if at all. Moms are the best. They sacrifice *everything* for their children, including their bodies. My own mother sacrificed for me; certainly my wife has sacrificed for our four children. Moms are always there, no matter what you need. But all that sacrifice—pregnancy, breast-feeding, months of getting up in the night, the erratic diet—has a price. Many women find that their bodies have been permanently changed by having children. They've become stretched out in some areas, droopy in others. They don't look or feel as good as they could.

That's where the Mommy Makeover comes in. Through safe, effective plastic surgery, we can restore a woman's body and reverse the effects of childbearing. To me, it's a great joy to be able to help a woman transform or renew her appearance. After all the sacrifices she makes in her life for her family, she *deserves* something for herself. To be a part of that change is awesome. And, in some small way, it makes me feel like I'm helping my own mother or my own wife when I help make another mom look better. I love to help moms achieve dreams they have been thinking about (and putting off) for a long time.

Here's a snapshot of one of my patients, Kristin. She was in her early 30s and the mother of two adorable young kids. She was physically in great shape, but two pregnancies and all that breast-feeding had permanently altered her body. Her breasts were deflated; she had a belly overhang that no amount of dieting and crunches in the gym could fix. She felt embarrassed and frustrated at how her appearance changed by having kids. She didn't mind the sacrifice, but Kristin really wanted her body back. She brought the idea of plastic surgery up with her husband, concerned that he might disapprove. To her surprise, he was all for it. That was all Kristin needed to call my office and make an introductory appointment.

Kristin went through with a Mommy Makeover that included a breast lift with conservative augmentation and a tummy tuck. After the surgery, Kristin was one of the happiest patients I have ever had. She was just ecstatic over her restored body. She healed up beautifully and very quickly. When I saw her in a follow-up visit, she had a new confidence and new vibrancy. Her self-image soared. She went to the neighborhood pool without reservation, she looked forward to shopping again, and the relationships in her life improved. It's what the Mommy Makeover is all about.

Every mom knows that having kids is a huge physical sacrifice. You're reminded of it every day when you look in the mirror. During pregnancy, your body expands—it changes and grows as your unborn baby matures. Your breasts get larger in preparation for breast-feeding. Your abdomen swells, the skin stretches, and you gain weight as the baby grows larger and you eat more to feed you both.

All this takes a toll on your body. Generally, after the baby is born, the abdominal area gradually shrinks back down and some, even most, of the extra baby weight comes off. When you stop breast-feeding (or if you didn't breast-feed at all), your breasts will gradually get smaller as well.

But nothing in your body fully returns to just what it was before pregnancy. And the more children a woman has, the more the physical changes are likely to be permanent. My wife likes to remind me that something "breaks" with each pregnancy. And she is right. As the baby grows, for instance, the fibrous band of tissue that runs down the middle of the abdomen can become permanently stretched out of shape. Many women end up with what some of my patients call a *dunlap*. (A strange Southern term for a Jersey boy like me. It means muffin top, pooch, or love handles when referring to the abdomen, as in "My belly has done lapped over my belt.")

A woman's breasts are permanently changed by pregnancy and breast-feeding. And that scientific paper I read as a young resident that claimed that breast-feeding had no effect on breast size and shape? Quickly debunked by my wife when I shared it with her after the birth of our second child. If I remember correctly, she threw that paper against the wall, stomped on it, and glared at me. After seeing countless patients in my practice, I *now* know that by the time a woman has had her second or third child, her breasts are often deflated and pointing south. Bulges, stretch marks, wrinkles, shape changes, drooping—no matter how hard you work out, no matter how diligently you diet, no matter how many expensive creams or products you use, things will never be quite the same as before.

All these changes and the continuing futility of the effort to recover from them can make a woman feel worn-out, unattractive, demotivated, and generally unhappy. Some women find that they have lost their self-confidence; others worry that they are less desirable to their partners; some describe feeling old before their time. And there are cases where the changes from childbearing can be physically uncomfortable or can interfere with a woman's day-to-day life activities.

Women put up with *a lot* during pregnancy, childbirth, and the aftermath. Morning sickness, heartburn, swelling, waddling, shortness of breath, changes in skin and hair, feeling "as big as a house" (per my wife), frequent trips to the bathroom, trouble sleeping at night, and restrictions on what to eat and drink. You do your best, eat well, avoid caffeine and alcohol, try to keep moving, and take naps when you can. Then the baby comes—and you are instantly turned into a milk factory, open and needed at all hours. And you are tired! Will you *ever* again have time for yourself? When is it mommy time?

After all this sacrifice, its impact on your physical and emotional well-being, your very sanity, perhaps it is time to consider something for *you*. Perhaps it's time to consider a Mommy Makeover. Let's take a look at what that means.

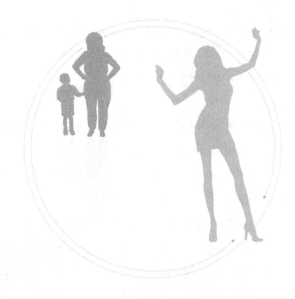

Chapter 2

WHAT IS A MOMMY MAKEOVER?

A Mommy Makeover is plastic surgery, also known as cosmetic surgery, to restore a woman's body after childbirth. A Mommy Makeover may include some or almost all of the following procedures:

- A tummy tuck to remove stretched-out skin, excess fat, and stretch marks in the abdomen. The procedure also tightens up the midline and can even reposition your belly button.
- Liposuction to remove stubborn fat in the midline, love handles, and sometimes the thighs and hips. We can also do liposuction in the bra strap area.

- Breast augmentation to restore the flattened upper area of the breasts and bring back your cleavage.
- A breast lift to raise sagging breasts and restore the nipples to their original position. We can also improve the appearance of the nipple and areola (the pigmented area around the nipple).
- Breast reduction to remove excess weight still trapped in your breasts.
- Labiaplasty to restore the vaginal area, tighten the excess tissue that may have been permanently stretched during pregnancy and the birthing process, and/or improve the appearance of the genital area.
- Eyelid lift to remove wrinkles and under-eye bags from all those sleepless nights with the baby.
- Other facial procedures, including Botox to help remove the elevens (vertical wrinkles between the eyes), crow's feet, and other wrinkles, or HA (hyaluronic acid) fillers (Voluma, Restylane, Juvederm) or fat transfers to improve the wrinkles around the nose, mouth, and lips and to restore fullness in cheeks.

We will discuss each of these procedures in more detail in later chapters. We will also cover skin-care concepts (safe to use while pregnant or breast-feeding—just in case), as well as some recommendations on the best food for your skin and how to avoid and treat stretch marks. But first let's talk more about the bigger picture of deciding whether a Mommy Makeover might be right for *you*.

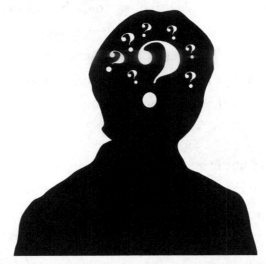

TELL ME, WHAT DON'T YOU LIKE ABOUT YOURSELF?

When a mom visits me in my office for the first time, we spend time talking about how she feels about her body right now:

- What parts do you like? Why?
- What are your areas of greatest concern? Why?
- How did you feel about your body before your first pregnancy?
- How has your appearance changed since?
- How would you like your body to be different in the future?
- Are you happy with the size and shape of your breasts?
- Is it time for the bigger breasts you have always wanted?
- Are you confident in tight-fitting clothes or being seen naked?
- Do you wear a bikini now? Will you in the future? What will that take?

Some women say they liked the way their breasts looked while they were breast-feeding. Now that they have stopped, they feel that their breasts look like "fried eggs" or "pancakes flopping on their chest." Some moms just want more fullness, others want a little more cleavage, and some want their nipples to stop "looking downward." It's all possible.

Some women come in and tell me, "I hate the way I look in jeans," or "I hate the way my belly hangs over," or "I want to get back into that bikini." Others just say, "I want to get rid of this extra weight." These concerns can be met too.

Of course, some want to restore both their breasts and their bellies.

One thing I've learned over my years in practice is that no two women will have the same desires or concerns. It's all a very, very personal and individual decision. I like to help my patients dream a little about where they see themselves after surgery: what they would like their results to be. That's where all the questions above come into play. As a surgeon, I can guide you through what is appropriate and safe, as well as what can be done in a single surgery versus multiple surgeries. As a patient thinks through the possibilities, I can help her process and envision what the end result could be. Then we can discuss what Mommy Makeover procedures are right for her.

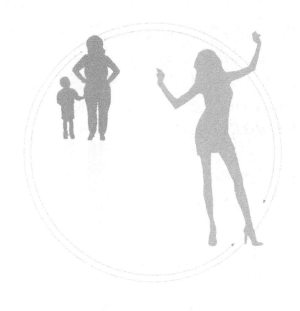

Chapter 3

IS A MOMMY MAKEOVER RIGHT FOR YOU?

Having dreamed the dream and seen the vision, there are now other questions to be worked through. Plastic surgery is a big decision, one you should not enter into flippantly. I work closely with my patients to help them distinguish the difference between their desires and what's appropriate and possible, to understand the benefits and some potential challenges that are in store for them.

- Are you ready mentally and emotionally for this change in your life?

- How do you feel about plastic surgery in general?
- Can and will you give yourself permission to actually have plastic surgery?
- Is the timing right? Do you plan to have more children?
- Is it safe? Can combination procedures be performed on you?
- How will you pay for it?

Let's take these one at a time.

MENTAL AND EMOTIONAL

Plastic surgery definitely has side effects—some good and some more challenging. We'll talk about these as you prepare for your Mommy Makeover.

Some points to consider:

- The transformation in your self-image—you'll feel more self-confident, leading to good things in your life, your career.
- The responses of those around you to your decision— some will celebrate with you, and some will question you.
- The potential impact on relationships—some will be pleased for you, some will be critical or even jealous, and some relationships may even be reinvigorated.

Are you mentally and psychologically prepared for making this significant change in your body? Are you ready for the compliments and the new wardrobe? Are you ready for the reactions of those around you? You need to mentally prepare for all the challenges and the victories that encompass a Mommy Makeover.

WHAT'S YOUR PERSPECTIVE ON PLASTIC SURGERY?

We've come a long way …

Plastic surgery is no longer something to be embarrassed about. Moms talk about it, work through their decisions openly, share their results, tell their friends. In fact, many of my patients come to me through referrals. They tell their friends, "I was where you are three years ago, and I finally decided to do it. I just wish I would have done it much sooner." People now don't worry as much about being thought of as vain or self-centered if they have surgery. Instead, they realize that they're doing something to make themselves feel better and look better as well. To me, that is a healthy approach to cosmetic surgery. (To see some of these results, visit my website www.musiccityplasticsurgery.com/galleries/)

I had one patient who was extremely shy and nervous. She was so embarrassed that she just closed her eyes during the preoperative photos. Shortly after surgery, her embarrassment vanished, and she asked, "Well, when are you going to use my pictures on your website? I've already told about five women to come see you." I remember thinking to myself, "What happened to the shy, demure girl that I met two months ago?"

PERMISSION: MAY I PLEASE DO THE MOMMY MAKEOVER? ASK *YOURSELF* FIRST

I see many mothers who feel guilty even considering doing the littlest things for themselves, let alone plastic surgery. It seems to stem from the inherent nature of moms to think of everyone else first and always put themselves last. Let me ask you: If all the logistics of childcare and household duties were met, all your questions answered, and all your concerns addressed (which I'll attempt to do throughout this book), will you *then* give yourself permission to have plastic surgery? Do you feel you're worth it? Only you can answer this question. But I say, if you are a mom who has sacrificed to carry a baby and has gone through the delivery process, you have more than earned it. And, as we all know, a mom's sacrifice doesn't just end with the delivery; it continues through the life of her child.

I have seen so many families blossom from having a mother who is happy and confident in herself. This surgery not only affects the individual woman but, like anything a mom does, can profoundly affect her entire family, too.

TIMING: MOMMY MAKEOVER NOW OR MOMMY MAKEOVER LATER?

When is the best time to do a Mommy Makeover? As I said before, plastic surgery isn't something to rush into. Many of the body changes that occur with pregnancy do improve quite a bit after child-birth, but it can take a while to lose the baby weight and get toned up. Some women I treat have thought about cosmetic surgery for years. When they're done having children, they come to me and say, "You know what? It's time. I am ready for this change."

We certainly want to be sure that all the hormonal changes of pregnancy and breast-feeding are done and you've given your body enough time to normalize as much as possible. This can take anywhere from three to six months after you've completed breast-feeding. Whether it's breast surgery or a tummy tuck, we want your body to have settled back into a normal pre-pregnancy state as much as it will. For facial work, it's best to wait until the baby is sleeping through the night and give your eyes a chance to recover. Botox can't be administered until you are finished breast-feeding. For labiaplasty, it's best to wait at least three, and preferably six, months to allow swelling to go down and things to return to a more normal state.

A Mommy Makeover has the best results when Mom has done all she can to get herself ready for it. That means losing as much of the excess baby weight as possible by following a healthy diet. It also means getting herself into the best physical shape she can. That doesn't mean training for a marathon in between diaper changes, but it does mean doing what you can to work some regular exercise into your life. When you've worked to lose weight and get fitter, we can then more easily see the areas that can't be fixed by diet and exercise alone. The better shape you're in preoperation, the quicker and easier you're going to recover, the less pain you're going to experience, and the better results you're going to get. We want to optimize it all!

A big factor in deciding when to have a Mommy Makeover is whether you plan to have more children. If you have a tummy tuck, being pregnant again could stretch out the area that is tightened in surgery. With the weight gain of pregnancy, it could even seem like fat has returned to areas that had liposuction. It's also possible that the tightened area of the midline could restrict the growth process of the baby as your pregnancy progresses. Many women worry that a breast lift and augmentation will affect their ability to breast-feed. While it is possible to have problems, we find that in almost all cases, the surgery doesn't cause any, and Mom can breast-feed successfully. If any problems do arise, they are usually minor and almost always go away over time.

The younger and healthier you are preoperatively, the easier time you will have with recovery postoperatively. While many objections can be made about why *not* to do it now, I believe in living life to the fullest.

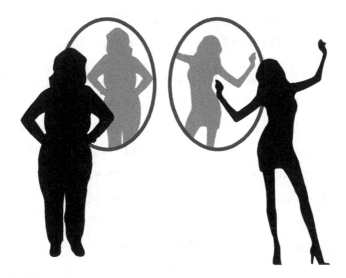

If you look at yourself in the mirror and don't like what you see, do something about it. There is never the perfect time to have surgery. Life happens. Kids will still have school, homework, after-school activities; the endless number of items on the to-do list won't go away. If you are anything like my wife, the allure of completing the unfinished projects stack will continue to drift away just out of arm's reach.

The timing of Mommy Makeover surgery involves many factors: the physical changes from pregnancy, your desire for more children, your age and overall health, and your life circumstances, which of course, include financial, too. We'll continue to cover the rest of these considerations in this book, but my overriding thought is if most of these line up—why wait? You deserve to enjoy a better body now. But let's not get ahead of ourselves. Let's delve deeper into some of the other concerns I have seen moms face when making these decisions.

SAFETY FIRST—IS A MOMMY MAKEOVER SAFE?

The usual procedures for a Mommy Makeover are very safe. (See Part 3 for specifics of the individual procedures. Obviously, it will be up to your board-certified plastic surgeon to determine your individual risks.) If you have a skilled surgeon working in a modern operating room, complications during the surgery are very rare. From my experience, most moms are relatively young and healthy without serious medical problems. And that's including the latest trend of current moms in their 30s and 40s. The thinking today is that 60 is the new 40. So 40 is really young—and so is 60! Those factors make the surgery and healing much easier on the body. A healthy mom can certainly go through several procedures at once safely and make a good recovery. This doesn't add much to the length of the surgery or the time you're under anesthesia. We jokingly ask our patients, "Why waste a good general anesthesia on only one surgery?" The additional pain and healing time isn't much greater either—approximately two to three weeks separately and only slightly longer when combined. Most prefer to just have that downtime once. Usually, there's also no long-term detriment to your system to undergoing the breast and belly procedures at the same time.

Many moms are surprised to learn this about a Mommy Makeover. Many come to the office with preconceived notions that only one problem can be fixed at a time due to the safety, pain, or recovery time. After we discuss it, however, most moms choose the combination Mommy Makeover. They understand that they're going to have to make a lot of arrangements for the household, children, meals, and so on—they'd rather have to do that just once. Plus, doing the procedures separately just means going through the preparation and downtime more often. And why pay the hospital operating room and facility fees more than once?

Advantages of Combined Procedures

- Single anesthetic (may be safer)
- Single downtime
- Similar pain
- Arrangements (kids, house, etc.) only once
- Potential savings (anesthesia and facility fees)

There are some situations where a Mommy Makeover may not be safe for you. Rarely, a patient has a serious disease like brittle diabetes, severe kidney or heart disease, or very high blood pressure; these are conditions that can cause problems with wound healing. The same is true if you're a smoker. I ask my patients who smoke to quit at least six weeks before surgery and to agree not to smoke again until they're completely healed.

The most common medical condition I see among my patients is actually a bit of depression. That's not unexpected in women who are tired out by pregnancy and childrearing and are feeling unhappy about all the changes in their body. I've found that a Mommy

Makeover does a huge amount to make depressed moms feel a lot better about themselves. It can really change their outlook not only about themselves but about their life in general. (More on this topic in Part 2.)

PAYING FOR YOUR MOMMY MAKEOVER—YOU'RE WORTH IT!

This is an area where many moms struggle—granting themselves permission to spend money on something they want. This is cosmetic surgery, not covered by health insurance. Any Mom can *always* find better uses for the money than on herself—something for the kids, family, house, etc.

A Mommy Makeover does cost real money, but it's not an indulgence or being selfish. It's a one time investment in yourself—one in which you'll reap the rewards for the rest of your life. It's not like a car, which eventually has to be traded in, or a house, where you have constant maintenance. A better way to look at this may be not "What does it cost" but rather, "How much is it worth to you?" How many times do you look in a mirror every day? And how many times do you think, *I wish I could get this taken care of?* How much is it worth to look in the mirror every time for the rest of your life and feel good about yourself? Would you pay a penny each time? If you would, then you've already more than covered your investment.

My office staff works with our patients to finance their surgery. There are many good options here. Some people put it on a credit card and get the bonus miles or points. Some specialized lenders will finance it—we can help set that up for you. The companies work with you on the repayment terms. We're also open to working out a payment plan with you. Because a Mommy Makeover is planned for and scheduled in advance, you know up-front what it will cost and when the payment is due. This cost includes surgery, follow-up, anesthesia, and facility fees. (To explore the financing option that works best for you, visit www.musiccityplasticsurgery.com/financing.)

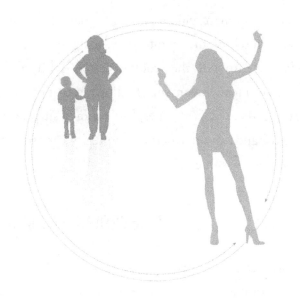

Chapter 4

LET'S TALK: DISCUSSING YOUR MOMMY MAKEOVER WITH YOUR SPOUSE

Talking about a Mommy Makeover with your partner may be a bit difficult. Sometimes Mom doesn't want to bring it up because she doesn't feel she deserves to have the money spent on her. Other times, she may be fearful that her husband might feel that way. If she does bring it up, her partner may be likely to respond with the dismissive, "You look beautiful to me just as you are."

Oftentimes, a woman will already have had the conversation in her head with her husband before broaching the topic with him. She's already come up with the problems or his rebuttals before they even talk. I encourage all women, on all matters, not to do this. We are men, true, and are jerks at times, but we may surprise you. In my experience, husbands and partners are typically very supportive once the woman raises the subject.

IT'S OKAY TO BE VULNERABLE WITH THOSE YOU LOVE

Many times, the hesitancy to bring up the Mommy Makeover doesn't involve money but other factors. By discussing areas that are bothering her, a woman becomes vulnerable and has to outwardly admit and verbalize that she isn't a perfect *super mom*. (As a medical doctor, I can assure you, this species does *not* exist.) She may feel like a failure because she can't get her body back in perfect shape. She can run the house, take care of the kids, and have a career, but she can't seem to take care of herself. Admitting this "defeat" (if it can be called that) can be difficult and embarrassing.

DON'T LET ANYTHING HAPPEN— HER SAFETY IS THE FIRST PRIORITY

Many women worry what their husbands or partners will think of them for considering cosmetic surgery. "Will he think I'm being stupid for being so vain? What will he think of implants? What are his thoughts on plastic surgery?" From our experience, these aren't the main issues. Most husbands' main concerns revolve around the protection of their wives. Truly, they want to make sure that their loved one will be safe going through these procedures and through the healing process. It's tough for men to watch our wives go through pain, for which there is nothing we can do. I hated watching my wife go through labor. I couldn't do anything about those pains, which I was reminded often that I caused. From our experience, we find that once a husband knows his wife will be taken care of and will remain safe, he is on board with the Mommy Makeover.

Sometimes, despite the factors listed above, the husband is still resistant to the idea of surgery, for whatever reason. I often ask the spouse to come in with his wife and meet with me for the consultation. That's very powerful. When a husband looks with his wife at before-and-after pictures or sees her try on breast implants and sees the big smile on her face, he's usually easily convinced. He also feels better when he gets all his questions answered and hears from me about how safe the surgery will be.

A few women come in and want to do it all totally privately. They won't tell their husband, sometimes because they think he won't approve; in some cases, they're about to get a divorce and want to have the Mommy Makeover paid for before that. But I also see women who want to surprise their husbands. Often their husbands are away for a long period on military duty or some other work assignment, so they can do it all without his ever knowing until he comes home to an exciting surprise. One of the most important things when considering a Mommy Makeover is that *you* have to be comfortable in what you're doing with *your* body. Your husband may or may not like it, but ultimately it's not for him, it's for you. It's for your confidence. It's for how you feel about yourself.

Not all my patients have partners, or if they do, the partner might agree to the surgery but not want to be very involved with it. Some women go at it alone, but often they come in with a friend for support.

I encourage this, because it's helpful to have someone to talk through the issues with and support you in your decision. In fact, sometimes a group of women will come in to support a friend and get interested in Mommy Makeovers for themselves. They let the friend be their test case. When they see that she comes through fine and looks great, they decide to go all in as a group. Sometimes women friends decide to go through it together. They can heal up together and keep each other company. They also understand and support one another in a way a man just can't. Sometimes friends decide to do the Mommy Makeover one after the other, and then it's just a question of them working out between them who gets to go first.

TEAMWORK: A MOMMY MAKEOVER IS A FAMILY AFFAIR

While each case is certainly unique, I believe the best Mommy Makeover is one that's a family adventure. Mom needs support during the lead-up to the surgery and during the recovery period afterward. The key is to be open and honest. Don't let your spouse/partner or kids (if they're old enough to understand) feel left out or uninvolved. (More on discussing the Mommy Makeover with your children in Part 2.) Cosmetic surgery can enhance your confidence and intimacy with your spouse. Just by discussing the possibilities of a Mommy Makeover, a new level of vulnerability can be explored and intimacy increased. Maintaining a high level of trust only increases the results.

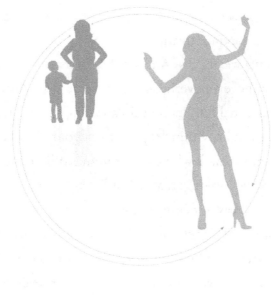

Chapter 5

WHAT A MOMMY MAKEOVER ISN'T

Having realistic expectations about your Mommy Makeover is crucial for being happy with the results, especially in the long run. It's important to know what a Mommy Makeover *can't* do for you.

- It *can't* save your marriage. If your marriage is already strained, going through the surgery won't help and might even put more stress on your relationship. I always discuss this aspect with my patients. I explain that at the end of the day, it's your body. If you're trying to look like the hot young secretary at his office, that won't happen. That's not a good motivation for surgery.

- It's *not* weight loss surgery. A tummy tuck is meant to remove an overhang, not remove large amounts of abdominal fat. Before I do a tummy tuck, I recommend that you be within 10 percent of your ideal body weight—that's where you're going to have the best results. Liposuction only removes small amounts of body fat in select areas. Of course, losing weight is easier said than done, and sometimes women will choose to go through the surgery a little bit before they get to that 10 percent ideal body weight level; some just can't ever get there. The results can still be good, if not excellent, and some patients are willing to accept that.

- It's *not* magic. You're trying to look and be the best that you can be. I can't turn you into somebody else.

- It *won't* turn the clock back 20 years. A Mommy Makeover can do a lot to restore your body to its pre-pregnancy shape and give you a more youthful appearance, but we can't make you look like you're a teenager again.

Mommy Makeover Readiness Quiz

Are you ready for a Mommy Makeover? Ask yourself these questions:

1. Do find yourself wondering, when is it *me* time?

2. Have you sacrificed *a lot* (or everything) for your family?

3. Do you feel like you lost *you* in caring for your children?

4. Does the thought of swimsuit season make you panic?

5. Is there a specific part of your body that bothers you? More than one part? Describe it.

6. Do you often use food to describe your various body parts? Muffin top? Sunny-side up breasts? Banana rolls?

7. Are you no longer in love with your love handles?

8. Have your breasts become deflated after breast-feeding?

9. Do you desire more cleavage?

10. Would you like to get rid of that pooch in your midsection?

11. Have you given yourself enough time after the baby to allow your body to restore itself on its own?

12. What's your exercise routine?

13. Are you planning more kids?

14. Can you arrange for the help you'll need during the recovery period? (We'll discuss specifics of this in the next chapter.)

Part 2

Okay, you've made your decision to go for it and proceed with your Mommy Makeover. Congratulations! Getting ready for your Mommy Makeover is just as important as the decision process and even the surgery itself. If you're well prepared, you'll get through the recovery period faster and with a lot less stress. In this section, I'll explain all the logistics of what you need to consider in advance.

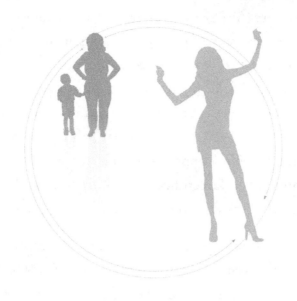

Chapter 6

CHOOSE THE RIGHT SURGEON

One of the most important decisions you have to make before having a procedure involves choosing a skilled and accredited plastic surgeon. This can be a bit confusing at first, because many doctors offer cosmetic procedures, and many consider themselves cosmetic surgeons. *However, a cosmetic surgeon and a plastic surgeon are not the same.* While it's true that all plastic surgeons are cosmetic surgeons, the reverse is not true. Plastic surgeons are trained in cosmetic and reconstructive surgery of the face and body (some are facial plastic surgeons only). A cosmetic surgeon may have a completely different kind of training. According to the American Board of Plastic Surgery (ABPS), a board-certified plastic surgeon must have a minimum of five years of residency training in all areas of surgery, including at least two years devoted entirely to plastic surgery. To become board-certified, the doctor then must pass comprehensive written (400 questions) and oral exams (where a panel of experienced expert surgeons grills you to make sure everything you do in and out of the operating room is appropriate, safe, and ethical). If you want to know more about the certification process or to see if a surgeon is board-certified, check the ABPS website at *www.abplsurg.org*.

Cosmetic surgeons are not necessarily plastic surgeons. Cosmetic surgeons are physicians of any specialty (like OB/GYN or emergency medicine) who have taken a course (often over just a weekend) in cosmetic surgery. So why does this matter? According to the Aesthetic Society for Aesthetic Plastic Surgery (ASAPS), physicians who call themselves cosmetic surgeons could be trained in any specialty, including a nonsurgical specialty; it is very unregulated. Just as you wouldn't want me, a plastic surgeon, to deliver your baby, you wouldn't want your OB/GYN, who calls himself a cosmetic surgeon, to do your tummy tuck. *If you stick only to plastic surgeons board-certified by the ABPS, you'll almost certainly end up in good hands.*

MORE THAN TEST SCORES

After confirming your surgeon is board-certified, you want to make sure that the surgeon has plenty of experience. As a general plastic surgeon, I am trained in plastic surgery from head to toe and am not confined to just one area of the body. You want to ensure your surgeon has dealt with issues at least as complex as your own: more complex, even better. There are some good ways to research this.

Websites

Browse through many websites to see which doctor's style makes you feel most comfortable. Look at the verbiage on the web pages to determine how they speak to their patients. Look at before and after pictures of the surgeon's work, and try to find a patient with similar characteristics to yourself.

References

Check online for patient reviews to ensure that the surgeon has plenty of satisfied patients. If possible, try to speak with former patients of the doctor you are considering. Be leery of surgeons who won't allow this—ask yourself if they are trying to hide something. Patients will likely give you the unabridged version of their experience. I am pleased to say that our patients give us very high marks. For me, there is no stronger compliment than a personal referral from a satisfied patient. I love it when some of my former patients take the opportunity to share their Music City Plastic Surgery experience with someone new and encourage them to experience us for themselves.

Consultation

The next step is having an initial consultation with the surgeon. This is when you and your surgeon get to know one another, face-to-face. When you first visit the surgeon, you shouldn't feel rushed or get the impression of a giant mass production machine. You should feel free to ask the surgeon anything, including details of his or her training and experience and what the surgery will cost. If you don't perceive a good connection with the surgeon or if you don't like any of his or her answers, it may be time to interview someone else. I often find that patients have talked to several doctors before deciding to work with me—and that's just fine. I especially like informed patients who have made a conscientious choice.

THE MUSIC CITY PLASTIC SURGERY EXPERIENCE

In my practice, I want to treat people exactly the way I would want my wife or mother to be treated. My goal is to deliver an unparalleled plastic surgery experience. I strive to empower my patients to look and feel their best in hopes that with this new confidence, they will make a positive impact on the lives and relationships of those around them. While you may initially feel a bit awkward and uncomfortable as we take our first steps, we hope you will quickly begin to feel you can trust everyone in the office as we aim to make your experience as positive and stress-free as possible. My staff and I want to overwhelm you with great care from the moment you call for the first time all the way through your last postoperative visit and beyond. It's an unwavering commitment to excellence to ensure we take care of your every need.

Mommy Makeovers involve very sensitive and private parts of the body. I make it a point to really take my time with all my patients and make sure they understand all of what they're about to do. The thorough education of my patients is an aspect in which I take great pride. I always talk to my patients as individuals first. I want to get to know them, where they're coming from, what's bothering them, and what they'd like to change (refer back to the list of questions in chapter 2). I listen very attentively to what my patients tell me. Only after establishing that relationship, that trust, do we get to the potentially awkward part of gowns and exams. And even that is dealt with in a slightly different manner; we use soft floor-length spa robes, not short, back-opened hospital gowns.

Most initial consultations take approximately an hour: slightly longer if we're sizing for breast implants. I like to truly get into the minds of my patients. I need to better understand *you* before I can try to understand the *parts* of you that you want to work on. With implants, for instance, I like you to try on a range of sizes, watching your reactions as we push the envelope on the extremes. I'll cover this in greater detail in chapter 15. While this approach may not seem to be the most efficient, I simply do not believe in rushing patients through a consultation in order to cram in as many as possible during a clinic period; I feel this gives me the best sense of who my patients really are and helps me understand their deepest dreams and desires. Only by spending so much time together can we jointly decide which path to take on *your* Mommy Makeover road to renewal.

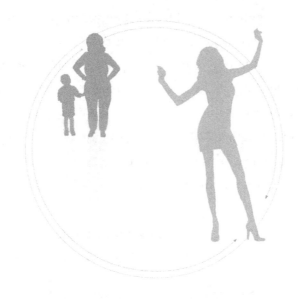

Chapter 7

EXPLAINING YOUR MOMMY MAKEOVER TO YOUR CHILDREN

S o how do you explain all this to your kids?

How do you tell them that Mommy won't be able to pick them up or cuddle them for a while? Depending on their ages, there may be other challenges to discuss: things like how to maintain a healthy body image for themselves (more on this below). This can all be a little tricky, because you want to be honest with your kids but not scare or worry them. We have found that what you say depends mostly on their age.

Many of my patients have kids in the five- to nine-year-old range. For kids at that age, you can tell them the basic limited truth. Say something like "Mommy is having a special mommy operation, and she won't be feeling well for a couple of weeks." That's usually about all young kids want or need to know. One of my patients told her eight-year-old daughter, "Mommy is going to have tummy surgery." When the girl asked why, she replied, "Because the doctor said so." The response at that point was simply, "Okay." A mother of all boys told them she was having "female surgery." As they ran out of the room to resume their sword fighting with a resounding, "Gross!" she knew that was all she needed to tell them.

Sometimes, however, limited information may not be enough. One patient recently told her daughter about her breast augmentation. The daughter expressed happiness for her mother but also concern. She wanted to know where they would "put her other breasts." You'll need to tailor the conversation to your children and your specific situation.

The concern about having the Mommy Makeover conversation with kids is one reason why some may decide to have the procedure sooner and not wait until later in life. One of my patients, Jennifer, a mom to a five-year-old boy and a seven-year-old girl, told me tongue-in-cheek, "I want to get this done before my daughter starts asking questions." Sometimes, it's less stressful and just easier to avoid the conversation.

MAINTAIN A POSITIVE BODY IMAGE IN YOUR CHILDREN

For older children, you might give more detail and explanation. In my view, we all need to be very careful about discussing plastic surgery with our children. As they grow up, we want them to have a positive body image. How their mom carries herself, how she responds to celebrities in popular media, and the language she uses to describe her own body have a strong impact on her children. Our kids need to know that cosmetic surgery isn't necessary to be attractive. They need to know that you're having surgery not to become a different person but instead to restore your body and to look as good as you feel.

The goal of a positive body image is particularly important for girls reaching their teens. As girls get older, they want to know more about your thinking and why you're doing a Mommy Makeover. Talk to your girls honestly, keeping in mind that you are an important role model for them. Here's how one of my patients explained it to her 13-year-old: "As a mom, I sacrificed to have children. My body has changed, and some of those changes I can't undo. What I've given to you I wouldn't trade for the world, but now I'm doing something for myself." I think that's a positive approach. I think it's fine and healthy for anybody, not just moms, to say, "Look, I've helped you out, and now it's time for me."

Boys can also be a little challenging when discussing medical matters. As a boy starts to mature, he is likely to start feeling protective of his mom and be more concerned with her safety. He may be interested in some of the details of the procedure or need more than a cursory explanation. This might allow him to feel some control over the situation or act as part of the "man of the family" even when Dad is standing right there. I am having fun watching this sort of maturity develop in my oldest son right now. When discussing body parts, we have always found it easier to use the anatomic terms in a matter-of-fact manner.

Sometimes, it may be easier for a son to hear the "doctor's pre-scription" of the procedure in order for it to be justified in his mind. That's exactly how it went for a 40-something mother of two who was having an eyelid lift. When she shared this news with her teenage children, her daughter greeted the news with squeals of excitement. "Good for you, Mom! I can't wait to see how you look!" Her son, however, was not convinced that he approved until she told him that "the doctor said this would only worsen over time." Then he supported her and remained right by her side for the duration of the postoperative recovery period. Now, many years later, this special bonding experience is one they treasure and frequently recount together.

Older teenagers can be an additional support system for Mom and the family, helping keep it all together and even instructing the other children. Sometimes when we challenge our children, we are pleasantly surprised at how they can rise to the occasion.

It is important to realize that how kids process things is not always what we would expect. I remember one story shared with me that involved a woman and her granddaughter. The grandmother had undergone a mastectomy many years prior for breast cancer and did not undergo reconstruction. Her young granddaughter one day, noticing the asymmetry and mastectomy scar when she saw her grandmother change clothes, innocently asked, "How old will I be when my booby falls off?"

Now having said all that, each situation, family, and child is different. Any number of responses can surface, some immedi-ately, others delayed. They may look like acting out rather than the concerns, fears, or questions they really are. Kids will want to know the impact on *them*. It may be fine that you're having surgery, but how will this affect me? (Okay. Husbands may be a little like this, too, myself included, but let's focus on the children for now.) Some concerns that may be thought and/or verbalized are:

How long will you be gone, Mommy?

Who will take care of me?

Will I stay home or go to school?

What will we eat?

And they might worry:

Is something wrong with you?

Are you sick? Are you going to die?

Will you be all right?

Will this happen to me, too? Now? When I grow up?

Kids should be encouraged to express their fears and ask their questions. Take your cues from them, being careful not to plant questions that haven't already occurred to them but answering thoughtfully those they ask. When Mom is out of commission, their world can be out of whack. As you anticipate your children's needs, they will feel more comfortable, and as Mom, you just might be able to recover a little more peacefully, knowing your children are more at ease with the whole situation.

This may also help your partner during your healing phase as well. It will be much easier to cut the kids some slack as they process and respond to your surgery if this perspective is kept in mind.

Generally, moms are pretty intuitive and will be able to infer the reaction of the children to hearing the news of her upcoming surgery.

With just a little forethought and preparation, and by anticipating questions and reactions to your surgery, both you and your partner are better prepared to help your children adjust in a healthy fashion to your Mommy Makeover.

And this is something I happily discuss and strategize with my patients to ensure comfort on every level.

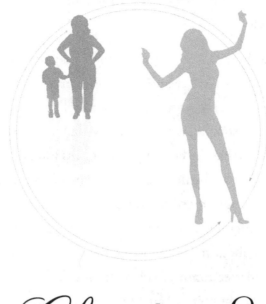

Chapter 8

DISCUSSING YOUR MOMMY MAKEOVER WITH FAMILY AND FRIENDS

Deciding to tell family and friends that you're planning a Mommy Makeover is another issue that often arises. And if so, then how? Today, plastic surgery is very common—it's not taboo, the secret it used to be. Let me reassure you that a lot of your family members and friends are going to respond by saying "Good for you!" as opposed to, "Oh my gosh, are you kidding me? You're going to have work done?" Many people see a Mommy Makeover as just another milestone, like having your tubes tied or your husband having a vasectomy.

Sometimes, however, family and friends may not see it this way or may even have negative views about plastic surgery. They may trigger some of your own fears or insecurities and tell you you're being vain or selfish—"You shouldn't spend money that way." We have found with our patients that the best response to this kind of objection is to explain the reasoning behind your decision. Help them understand the *why* behind your procedure. Instead of just saying, "I want fuller breasts," try telling them how the results will make you feel. "I really miss how I felt about my body before having kids, and having fuller breasts and a flatter tummy will make me feel more confident; it will be fun to go shopping again." Instead of saying, "I want to look younger," perhaps you can say, "I want my face to look as youthful as I feel." In general, those who love us want us to be happy— and won't begrudge us regaining confidence. The reasons behind your decision may help them to understand your deeper motivation and will, hopefully, help them to respect your personal decision. Make sure they understand that sharing with them means that you want them included in your life and your decisions (but you really don't need their approval).

Many times, the negative reaction comes from concern for your safety:

- Who's going to look after your children if something goes wrong?
- What if you choose the wrong size?
- Will you look fake afterward?
- Will you still look like yourself?

By performing your own initial research on the procedures (risks of surgery, rate of complications, etc.) and working out your own feelings about these versus the benefits of surgery before talking to them, you will be better prepared to reply to their concerns.

And, of course, we will talk all this through during our consultation as well. Having a list of objections that might be raised, with answers prepared, when you present your decision will go a long way toward alleviating their concerns more easily and softening their responses.

Please recognize that you may not be able to convince everyone that this is a good decision for you. Remember when you told family members what the baby's name would be? Some loved it, some hated it, but *everyone* had an opinion. That's the nature of families and friends. Just remember that none of them have actually walked in your shoes.

Also keep in mind the generation you are addressing. From some of the older folks, you may hear comments that sound grumpy and judgmental. "Well, *I* never had plastic surgery and I managed just fine." Definitely, perspectives change from one generation to the next, as do medical advances and technology. It doesn't mean you aren't strong and capable if you have a makeover. It doesn't make you a failure as a mom or as a woman.

As this can be an emotionally charged issue for any mother, we recommend you choose carefully with whom you share your decision. I encourage my patients to start with someone who will be more positive and supportive and use that conversation as a sort of dress rehearsal to gain confidence for dealing with those people you know will be difficult. This can be the practice run to get your *spiel* set.

If some people persist in giving you a hard time about the surgery (or you pretty much know they will), it might be best to avoid them until after you've healed. While this approach brings up potential feelings of distrust and betrayal, it might be best, especially in the immediate postoperative setting, when you're emotionally most fragile. (More on this below in the Emotional Roller Coaster section.) With my patients, we try to explore the relationship of concern and determine if it's better to ask for forgiveness instead of permission or to *tell, don't ask* first in order to include them in the process. Obviously, each case is dealt with individually.

That brings up another obstacle that might need to be hurdled when considering a Mommy Makeover. Some people may assume that having plastic surgery, losing weight, working out, and getting in shape means that marital problems exist and you are trying to compete for the attention of your husband. I almost feel these accusations are not worth a response. But a short explanation of how you are doing this for *you*, explaining your *why* behind the surgery, should quell these negative assumptions.

Because surgery is stressful in and of itself, I encourage you to seek out people who will be understanding and helpful. Remember, you're doing this for you. You're an adult woman and a mother— one who can (and does) make important decisions on her own. The positive effects of the surgery can far outweigh any of the pushback you might get.

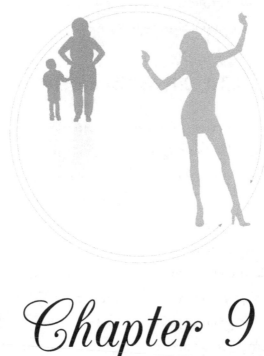

Chapter 9

PLANNING FOR YOUR
MOMMY MAKEOVER

I f you're a typical Mommy Makeover patient, you have at least one young child, a house, a job (in or out of the house), and probably a spouse or partner to think about as you plan for the surgery and your recovery. The most crucial point I have to make here is this: You have to think about *yourself* first during this time. For some (okay, many) women, setting up that *me time* can be a real mental and emotional struggle. This is often difficult, as moms are used to putting family first. They feel so guilty about taking any time for themselves. But it's extremely important to realize that you need to take enough *you* time in order to prepare and let yourself recover fully.

LET IT GO: PREPARING IN ADVANCE

Let's look at a time line for a typical Mommy Makeover surgery. Once you decide that you want to proceed, we usually schedule the surgery for a few weeks out. That gives you enough time to get a preoperative checkup by your primary care physician, organize payment, and get your recovery plan in place. You need to have someone nearby to help you with personal care and childcare for at least a week, preferably longer. You'll need to make arrangements at your workplace to be out for a couple of weeks and to get your home prepared in advance. Ideally, you'll want to clean the house, do the laundry, stock the fridge, put the takeout menus by the phone, arrange car pools, make lists and calendars, and get everything set up as far in advance as you can.

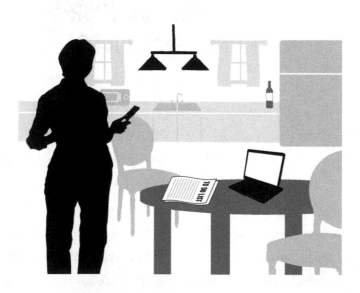

While you are recovering, set your expectations appropriately. Don't set yourself up for failure. Things are *not* going to go perfectly—no matter how much planning was done ahead of time. If you have kids, you're used to plans going awry—there are some days when you're falling back on plan D or E, not just plan B, before lunchtime. While you're recovering, the house will probably not be spick-and-span, the kids may run out of clean clothes. (Do you think they *really* mind wearing the same underwear three days in a row?) Their meals might not be ideal; playdates may have to be skipped (or done at someone else's house). This is not the time to be dragging loads of laundry back and forth or running the vacuum cleaner. All that stuff can wait. It really can. Trust me—I'm the father of four children and am married to another doctor. I have had to take over when my wife is on call—and we all survived!

Let it go! If the kids end up eating pizza every night for a week—Ha! They're smiling! In our house, my sons and I have a "man's meal" on nights my wife isn't there. Pizza, hot dogs, burgers, not a vegetable in sight (bachelor and little boy food!). Now, even when their mother is with us, they'll often request a "man's meal."

OUTTA SIGHT, OUTTA MIND

Here's another suggestion: avoid the chaos altogether. The messy house and the status of the kids tend to be the main reasons why many of my patients escape to a hotel for a few days after the surgery. If Mom can't hear the chaos of her children being children, Dad being Dad, and can't smell the smoke or that strange aroma emanating from the kitchen, she won't be tempted to act like Mom and get up and fix things. This option has become hugely popular among moms—we now have special accommodations (with the rare addition of nursing care) at a few local hotels for our postoperative patients. A beautiful room, no noise, room service, no temptations to get out of bed and do the laundry or feed the kids and pick up toys. And no guilt from staying in bed all day if you can't hear the kids in another room. Outta sight, outta mind means better recovery.

Mom, you've done all you can to arrange things in advance. Now, it's time to let others do for you. Just remove yourself from the situation (either physically or mentally or both) and concentrate on yourself. Nobody is starving … really!

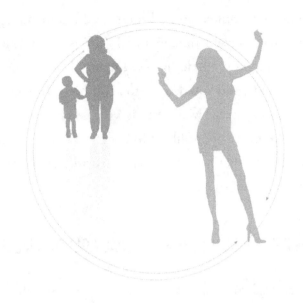

Chapter 10

RIDING THE EMOTIONAL
ROLLER COASTER

It's not uncommon for my patients to go on an emotional roller coaster ride as the surgery date approaches. Especially the night before, they may think, "Why am I doing this surgery? I've got kids. I've got a husband I need to live for. What if something goes wrong? I'm doing all of this for vanity's sake. I don't need fuller breasts. I don't need a flatter tummy. I don't need this flab of skin cut off. This is just silly."

Feeling anxious, guilty, and a little scared before an operation is perfectly natural. Second thoughts and doubts are normal. But try to remember that you are doing this for *you*. You've sacrificed your body for your kids, and you deserve to get it back. It helps to remind yourself that a Mommy Makeover is very, very safe. As I tell my patients, you're much more likely to get into a car accident on the way to the hospital than you are to have any problems during or after the surgery.

ANOTHER RIDE ON THE EMOTIONAL ROLLER COASTER

The emotional roller coaster ride continues with the aftereffects of surgery. You've got your new body, and you're ready to enjoy it, complete with the showers of compliments you will be hearing. But you might also be wondering, "How is my husband going to view me? I'm like a new person. Is this going to be good or bad?" For what it's worth, I have not had a single husband complain about the changes I helped make in his wife. Many times, it can reinvigorate their intimacy because of the added confidence the surgery can provide.

In the early postoperative period, emotional mood swings and short-term depression (or unmasking of subclinical depression) are common. Often this will manifest itself as tiredness, crying spells, and feeling "just not yourself." During the healing phase, you can go in a flash from being ecstatic about your surgery to crying hysterically for no apparent reason. Your emotional swings might remind you of when you were pregnant! As your surgeon, I can assure you this is perfectly natural—your emotions will soon return to normal.

But let's take a minute to explore why this happens.

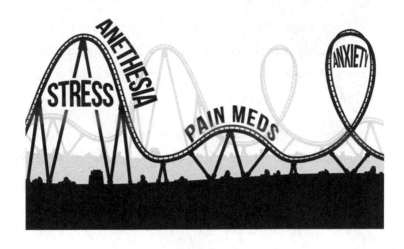

Although it's difficult to point to a single exact cause, many factors exist to build this emotional roller coaster. Surgery is a significant physical stress to your body, general anesthesia is used, narcotic pain medications are prescribed, and steroids may be used—all of which can throw off your hormone balances. Pain may interfere with sleeping and deplete your body's reserves, leaving you feeling tired and worn down. I believe you heal more quickly when you are not in pain because your body devotes the resources to healing and not fighting pain, so I encourage use of the pain medications, at least in the first few days. However, the anesthesia and pain medications can also alter sleep patterns. As any mom remembers from the early times of her children's lives, life becomes a lot more difficult when you are sleep deprived.

Most moms tend to be dynamic individuals, often "going" at all times. The elevated endorphins they are used to having from frequent workouts and high activity levels are reduced or nonexistent in the recovery phase, when Mom has to be uncharacteristically still. Many moms have difficulty in this unstructured healing time and get antsy to do something.

Stress has a *huge* role in how you deal with the postoperative period. We already mentioned the physical stress of surgery, but the mental stress of the impending surgery, and then waiting for the final outcome, play into your emotions as well.

Often with surgery, especially facial surgery, you may look worse before you look better. Seeing the swelling, bruising, and temporarily raised or reddened scars may leave Mom second-guessing why she voluntarily chose this. Anxiety works negatively in this situation. Anxiety about the results, about taking time for yourself, about being so behind in terms of your "job" as mom (the house is a mess, the kids are out of control, etc.), about being alone to fend for yourself if your husband has returned to work, about returning to your outside-the-house job sooner than you may feel ready for … the list can go on and on.

PUTTING THE BRAKES ON THE EMOTIONAL ROLLER COASTER

While these stressors are very real, the important thing to understand is that they can be minimized with a little planning and preparation. This emotional roller coaster often ends on its own, with just a little time.

Here are a few suggestions:

- Get outdoors—When able, try to spend a few minutes outside in the sunshine.
- Shower—Typically, a shower is allowed after two days. This goes a *long* way toward patients feeling themselves again.

- Eat healthy—Fruits, vegetables, and good protein intake speed recovery and provides your body with antioxidants to fight off stress.
- Enjoy friends—Surround yourself with positive people (see above), and avoid the negative ones.
- See your doctor—Schedule a visit to your plastic surgeon. Sometimes my words of encouragement can help alleviate the anxiety. Let me be your cheerleader.
- Use your computer responsibly—There's a lot of junk health information on the Internet. Visit ASPS, ASAPS, or www.realself.com for some positive feedback and stories about plastic surgery.

Remember the time frame for healing from surgery. Many times, full results are not appreciated for a few months. Give your body the chance to heal before you second-guess your decisions. We'll discuss the specifics of each procedure in the following chapters so you will be well prepared and informed when it's time for your surgery.

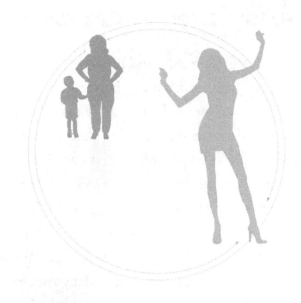

Chapter 11

The downtime from the surgery will generally last between two to three weeks—*and you need to take that time to fully recover.* It's extremely important not to force yourself back into that full-time, unpaid job of being mom too soon. If you do, you can definitely damage your results, have a lot more pain, and cause some long-term complications. The breast implants can move and shift around; you can stretch and/or tear the repair, especially with a tummy tuck, or cause the implant to come barreling out. Yikes!

PLAN SURGERY FOR WHEN HELP IS AVAILABLE

Along with arranging for child and household care, you will need some assistance of your own during the recovery period. That's a reality you need to plan for carefully. A lot of my patients arrange to do their Mommy Makeover during a slow time at work for them or their husbands. I operate on a lot of teachers over the summer or the holiday break, for example. Some of my patients have seasonal businesses and do the surgery in their off-peak period. I had one patient recently who saved up some extra vacation time for her surgery. When she went back to work, everyone said to her, "You look great! Your vacation must have been awesome!" Many spouses arrange to take a few days off to help out. That's why we do a lot of surgeries on Tuesday or Wednesday—the spouse takes a few vacation days and can also be home to help through the weekend.

Especially during the first days of your recovery period, you need an adult nearby to help you with things like getting out of bed, going to the bathroom, and getting dressed. If you've had a tummy tuck, for instance, one of the challenges is getting in and out of bed properly. We teach you how to do it so you don't strain, but having some help is still very important. If you've had breast work done, your chest muscles will be sore and you won't want to use them much. You might also have a drain in place in your abdomen or chest for a few days. That takes a little management. After surgery you'll also be wearing a surgical garment to hold things tightly in place. Getting that on and off is a bit of a challenge at first—you'll want to have someone help you. It also may be the time to consider hiring help, even if it's only in the short-term: babysitters, dog walkers, house cleaners, etc.

While you're recovering, you can't lift anything heavy, including a baby or toddler. You also won't be all that quick on your feet, so you'll have trouble running after the kids. While you're taking pain medications, you're not allowed to drive; once you're off the meds, driving may still be mildly uncomfortable for a while. If you do any of these things, you might hurt. To me, these are reminder pains that say, "Okay, I shouldn't be doing this. I need to slow it down."

If your spouse can't help much, this may be the time to ask friends and family members to pitch in. I say this with a little hesitation, though. Think this through carefully and be choosy about whom you invite. You want this time to be restful, not more stressful because someone "other" is in the house. You want it to be someone both you and your kids (and your husband) are completely comfortable with and can communicate clearly and honestly with. Remember that your emotions (and those of the kids) can be a bit on edge; be sure that your helper is someone that you can all feel supported by, not someone who might present additional challenges of their own.

We have found that the best people for this type of support are people who already know you and your family well (though hiring a private nurse just to take care of you isn't a bad idea either). You won't mind if they see you at your worst (physically and emotionally), when you haven't taken a shower and you're kind of groggy and grumpy. You also won't mind them seeing the house a mess and feel embarrassed or stressed to keep up appearances. Choose those who are most likely to step up and help out when you are most vulnerable.

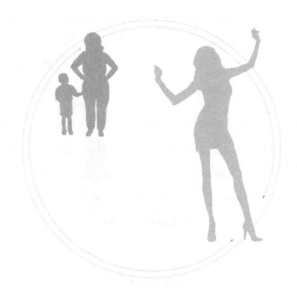

Chapter 12

YOUR MOMMY MAKEOVER
FOR THE LONG-TERM

No matter how skillful your surgeon is, no plastic surgery truly lasts forever. Gravity always wins, and your genetics play a big role in this as well. But there's a lot you can do to preserve your Mommy Makeover results over the years. Your lifestyle matters.

Remember that your Mommy Makeover isn't weight loss surgery. You'll want to aim for maintaining your normal weight or close to it. We want you to continue to exercise and avoid big weight fluctuations; this is a sound goal whether you have had surgery or not but even more important to maintain your surgical results. You don't want to gain weight and then crash diet it off. That's not good for your body in general, but it's also going to stretch out the skin in your abdomen and breasts.

Family history plays a role here, too. If your mother or father has really thin, wrinkly, or droopy skin, that can play into how your Mommy Makeover looks in 20 years. Surgery is one component to this. Genetics and lifestyle matter, too, and always will. That part is up to you. But if you're like many of the other moms I know, you can do it!

Are you prepared for your Mommy Makeover? Yes? Let's look in more detail at what each procedure involves.

Part 3

PROCEDURES

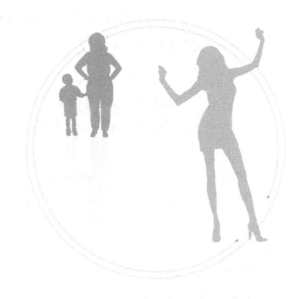

Chapter 13

TUMMY TUCK

The kids are in bed, and the kitchen is cleaned up. It's finally time for a few minutes of peace and quiet. You head to the shower and sigh as the water rushes over you; you relax and breathe. As you step out of the shower and reach for your towel, you catch a glimpse of yourself in the mirror—and you wonder out loud, "Whose belly is that, anyway?"

A growing baby can really wreak havoc on the abdominal area during pregnancy. The muscles and the skin stretch out; stretch marks may appear. And while the size of your tummy certainly goes down after giving birth, there are plenty of daily, visible reminders of what your body has just experienced.

After carrying a baby, the rectus abdominis muscles (your six-pack) can be permanently stretched out of place as well. They should face forward, but pregnancy, especially if you gained a lot of weight, can stretch out the tough band of fibrous tissue that runs down your midline (think of the row of buttons on a button-down shirt), causing the muscles to be shifted off to the side. When that band is stretched, it doesn't usually snap all the way back after the baby is born. (Think about when your son stretches out the neck of his T-shirt. Even after washing, it never really tightens back up.) The result is that "pooch" you see when you turn sideways. Instead of your old flat tummy, you look a little thicker from front to back. You can suck it in and try to hold it; you can do crunches in the gym religiously every day. You won't be able to tighten that fibrous connective tissue back down on your own.

Pregnancy also stretches the skin of the abdominal area, often beyond the point of repair. The skin is saggy, wrinkled, and may have some stretch marks. My patients call it "prune belly," an "apron," or "muffin top." The belly button is widened (remember how it stuck out during the last couple months of your pregnancy?) and may even be pointing south. Stretch marks happen because your body has expanded faster than your skin can. The elastic fibers below the skin break, causing reddish streaks. They may fade a bit after the baby is born, but they're there for good. Dieting, exercise, and expensive creams alone just can't return your skin to its original condition.

This is where you begin to consider the tummy tuck (abdomino-plasty). It will give you a flatter, tighter abdomen and will remove some or all of the stretch marks. You might even choose to combine it with a bit of liposuction (see chapter 14). The pooch is gone, the skin is tightened, the belly button is restored, and the muscles become visible again—wow!

Tummy Tuck Readiness Quiz: Are You Ready?

Have you lost most or all of your pregnancy weight?

Are you within 10 percent of your ideal body weight?

What have you done to get back into shape?

Do you have plans to have more children?

Did you have a Cesarean birth (C-section)?

Have you had any other surgery on your abdomen?

The first thing to note is that a tummy tuck is not weight loss surgery. As a general rule, I like moms to wait at least six months to a year after their last pregnancy and to be back to as close to normal as possible before we perform the surgery. In some cases, the tummy tuck can be just the motivator you need to get serious about losing weight. A body that is closer to its previous normal as a result of exercise and a healthy diet is one that will benefit most (and heal and recover more quickly) from the surgery and experience the best results. If you plan to have more children, this may not be the right time. We can discuss the issues in a consultation, but, in general, it is best to wait. If you had a C-section or have had other abdominal surgeries, we will need to take that into consideration as we plan.

Removing old scars and working around scar tissue needs to be part of our plan.

THE TUMMY TUCK EVALUATION

We start with an office evaluation to assess your abdominal skin and fat, determine if there are any stretch marks or other scars on your abdomen, and feel along the midline to identify any widening that needs to be tightened. I will use the "pinch test" (it doesn't hurt!) where I "pinch an inch" of skin and fat to see what can be removed. I will assess how you carry your fat and the degree of your skin's stretchiness to determine how it can move (and how much can be removed) during surgery.

Women tend to carry more fat externally, away from their internal organs under the skin (subcutaneous fat) as opposed to inside the body around the organs (known as visceral fat). Men usually have their fat stored as visceral fat under their muscles. That is why men tend to have a "beer gut" or a "barrel shape" that is solid when you push on it. The muscle is strong, and the fat is internal. For women, a tummy tuck can work very well because we can easily reach the external fat under the skin and remove it.

Everyone has *some* internal visceral fat. We can't remove that, but the plication (tucking) to tighten the midline acts like a corset and pushes that fat back into your body. When that happens, the overall thickness of your body from front to back is decreased. A side note here: If you have a lot of visceral fat, it's like trying to put a beach ball on your tummy and button your shirt over it as tight as you can get it. It just can't be compressed that much; it pushes back—and that's not pretty. The only way to reduce your visceral fat is to work it off with cardiovascular exercise and diet. Visceral fat is also associated with health problems, including type 2 diabetes and heart disease. Doing what you can to get rid of it is important.

I will evaluate your midline and see if there is any unremitting widening from pregnancy. The fibrous band that runs down the center of your abdomen, when widened, is called a diastasis recti. This vertical bulge pushes out and makes you appear thicker and heavier from front to back.

Finally, we will assess your sides, those love handles that many of us don't love so much. I will determine if you're a good candidate for combined liposuction (lipoabdominoplasty) in a single surgery or liposuction performed at a later time in a separate surgery.

Once we've completed the full assessment, I can determine if a standard tummy tuck is necessary or if a mini tummy tuck might suffice. The main difference between the two has to do with the length of incision and whether or not we reposition your belly button. The mini procedure has a smaller incision but also has smaller results. Since the belly button (umbilicus) sits on a stalk and is tethered to your strength layer underneath the skin, we can only pull downward so far without releasing it. The mini tummy tuck only cuts out a small ellipse of skin and fat below the belly button. The standard tummy tuck can reposition the belly button and, therefore, remove significantly more skin and fat from the abdominal region. This is a decision we can make together with the information from your evaluation.

THE TUMMY TUCK SURGERY

The first step in the surgery is to release the belly button with an incision. Here, the widened, stretched-out belly button can be tightened up by positioning the incision inside the circle of the umbilicus, thereby making the overall circumference of the opening smaller. Think of a black-eyed Susan flower. The dark part in the middle is the belly button, and the stalk extends deep to the skin and fat. The flower is incised around the edges, and the stalk is dissected out to its base. The "stalk" of the belly button is released and awaits repositioning.

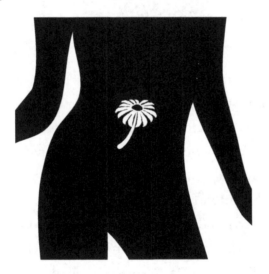

Next, a suprapubic incision that hides beneath the bikini line is made down to the muscle layer and extends in a gentle curve up toward each hip bone. This exposes a football-shaped area of skin and fat to be removed (the inch we previously pinched). The dissection continues past the belly button stalk, freeing enough tissue so it can be pulled down toward your toes, like a window shade. The rectus plication is performed next by tightening the widened fibrous band, reorienting the six-pack muscles, and then repositioning your smaller, more youthful-appearing belly button. The previously stretched-out, wrinkly football of abdominal skin and fat is punted from your body, and the incisions are closed.

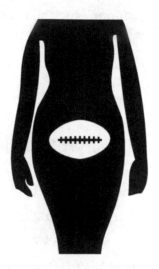

If you are also having liposuction, we do that before we close the incisions. This is a good time to do liposuction for those love handles on the hips because we already have access; we can do better contouring without making additional incisions. The liposuction doesn't add very much time or much risk to the surgery, when performed appropriately. About one-half to three-quarters of my patients choose to do liposuction with their tummy tuck (more about this in the next chapter).

When you visit my office for an evaluation, I'll illustrate these procedures using a button-down shirt. The shirt button directly overlying the belly button marks the incision site for belly button release. The larger incision is where the shirt tucks into pants. I dissect up under the shirt toward the rib cage. Once that is complete, the "internal corset" of the rectus plication is performed. Next, I pull the shirt down, and any bunched-up excess is excised and thrown into the trash. The belly button is repositioned in a more youthful and vertical position, and the lower incision is closed. Voilà! A smoother, flatter, younger tummy!

From start to finish, a tummy tuck takes anywhere from two and a half to four hours. If your overhang is small, the surgery can be even shorter. Liposuction to the love handles adds about 30 minutes to the procedure.

AFTER THE TUMMY TUCK SURGERY

A tummy tuck is an outpatient procedure; only rarely would you have to spend the night in the hospital. I'd much rather send you home than subject you to the risk of a hospital-acquired infection and to the interruptions to your rest (for example, a nurse waking you up in the middle of the night to ask how you're sleeping). You will be much happier at home in a familiar setting.

A tummy tuck is a very safe procedure and generally goes very smoothly. If you're young and healthy, the risk of complications is low. We do, however, carefully monitor for blood clots in the veins of your calf muscle (deep vein thrombosis or DVT). While this likelihood is minimal (less than 1 percent and most commonly occurring between 5 and 14 days postsurgery), if it does happen, it can be very dangerous. The best way to prevent DVT is to use these muscles to circulate blood by walking. I insist that all my patients walk a short distance, with assistance, the night of the surgery and a minimum of three times a day thereafter.

The recovery period after a tummy tuck lasts about two weeks. The first night after the surgery is usually not too difficult because you will still be enjoying the effects of the anesthesia and the numbing medications I use for the incision. Days two, three, and maybe even four will likely be the most uncomfortable. You can expect some pain, and you probably won't be very excited about getting out of bed much. You still *must* get up and walk, however, to prevent a blood clot. Pain medication can help quite a bit during this period. I typically send you home with these, along with muscle relaxants and anti-nausea medication, which can help prevent the unhappy experience of vomiting with sore tummy muscles. If you are taking these medications, be very cautious and ask for help when you are getting up.

You can eat normally as soon as you feel like it. Most patients start off with bland food—crackers and ginger ale are recommended. Pain medications are notorious for causing constipation, so you may want to include salads and other vegetables for the fiber, or try some over-the-counter medications to help with this. On the flip side, you may find that you need to urinate more than usual for the first few days after surgery. That's a good thing—and will also get you out of bed regularly.

I allow my patients to shower after two days. We have found this goes a *long* way toward helping you feel human again, which speeds the recovery along.

As you continue to recover, you will continuously be wearing a spandex-type compression garment that fits like a body suit. For the best results, it is really best to wear this 24-7 (except when showering) for the next six weeks.

Getting in and out of bed seems to be one of the biggest challenges during recovery because of the soreness in your abdominal muscles. We'll teach you how to log roll onto your side and push up with your arms to get in and out of bed. It's the best way to avoid straining the muscles and to minimize the discomfort.

For the first few days, you will have some temporary drains in place to remove the expected fluid buildup and prevent pressure on your incisions. Whenever I move skin and fat to a new place (remember the "window shade"), it tends to rub against the other tissues and secrete fluid. This is absolutely normal and expected. We'll teach you how to easily manage these drains while at home.

During the postoperative healing period, the skin between your belly button and your pubic area may feel numb. The nerves in that area have been dissected from underneath and stretched. The changes in nerve sensation usually return to normal within a few years.

Within a week of the surgery, I will see you in my office for a postoperative visit and to remove the drains. Once the drains are out, you can gradually resume your normal activities. For the next three months, you should avoid straining the abdominal area—no heavy lifting, crunches, or core workouts. I normally release my patients to resume activity and exercise (with the exceptions mentioned above) within two weeks from surgery. It's okay to resume having sex whenever you feel up to it; you may need to be creative in position-ing to avoid strain and discomfort. As always, I recommend that you listen carefully to your body as to how intense your activities might be.

The scar from the tummy tuck heals up quickly and becomes almost invisible within a couple of years. It will never go away completely but will definitely fade down to where it is very close to normal-colored skin, perhaps with just a slight discoloration. The scar is almost entirely hidden below the pantie line. To minimize the scarring, we ask that, at the three-week point, you start lightly massaging the area. I'm often asked for products to use on the scarring. Options include vitamin E, cocoa butter, coconut oil, body lotion, and baby oil, but the only thing that has actually been proven to help is a silicone-based scar cream. Plain old Vaseline seems to work really well, too. The real key is to use something that lubricates the skin as you massage it—and to be gentle with the scarred area to avoid damaging it. I have seen allergic reactions to antibiotic ointments or vitamin E. When I see scars that have turned red, I always ask first, "What are you putting on it?"

Poor wound healing is another minor hazard. In almost every case, the wound heals quickly and cleanly. A preexisting health problem like diabetes can cause a patient to heal more slowly. In rare cases, the midline part of the incision, where the tension is greatest, can become infected, or the skin can break down and cause wound healing complications. Sometimes we see poor scarring. For reasons we don't really understand, some people form keloids, a tough, thick scar that rises up above the skin. Sometimes the scar is asymmetric (or "catawampus" as they say in Mississippi). This usually happens if the abdominal flap is pulled down unevenly, too tight on one side, or not tight enough on the other. We can sometimes see "dog ears," little overhangs or puckers in the skin near the far ends of the incision. These often go away within a few months. If necessary, we can easily do a little scar revision in the office under local anesthetic.

YOUR TUMMY TUCK OVER TIME

Almost everybody heals up quickly from a tummy tuck; the scar gradually fades away to near invisibility. In the long term, the major concern is weight fluctuation, which could stretch out the skin in the abdomen all over again and could create more stretch marks (sometimes worse than before, as your skin is tighter from your surgery). However, if you keep your weight in the normal range and stay reasonably fit, the results should stand up well, with no major risk of drooping or stretching.

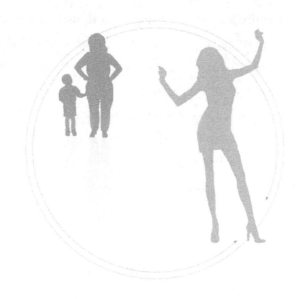

Chapter 14

LIPOSUCTION

Your baby has come, you've stopped breast-feeding, and you've spent the last six months or more losing weight and working out (in your spare time). You're close to your pre-baby weight or even back at it, but despite your best efforts, you've still got those annoying love handles at your waist, a pooch on your belly, and that muffin top thing above your favorite jeans. Don't blame yourself. Many times, those stubborn areas harbor excess fat that is unreachable by diet and exercise alone. Sometimes, you just can't tone those bumpy spots away. But you don't need to live with them! You can choose to get rid of them with liposuction.

Liposuction (also known as lipoplasty or liposculpture) can make a big difference in giving you back your trim, pre-baby body. I remove small amounts of subcutaneous fat in specific locations in order to smooth and shape your appearance. I can't just suck away all your excess weight. In fact, I ask my patients to be within 20 percent of their optimal weight before I perform the procedure—it's not weight loss surgery or a substitute for weight loss. And it's important that you get to that weight through healthy eating and exercise, not crash dieting.

WHAT IS LIPOSUCTION?

Liposuction is the part of a Mommy Makeover that will remove those love handles and reduce the abdominal and hip fat that isn't removed with the tummy tuck. For moms who don't have widened abdominal muscles or a lot of stretched-out skin from pregnancy and don't need a tummy tuck, liposuction can be done on its own to good effect. Liposuction can also reduce areas of fat around the bra straps as well as remove fat from the thighs and buttocks. It is also fairly effective for getting rid of cellulite in the thighs.

Liposuction means, literally, fat removal by suction, performed using specialized techniques and protocol. Several types of liposuction techniques and equipment are in use today, with various names or acronyms that seem to improve their marketability, not necessarily the results. The current most popular are laser, power-assisted, or ultrasonic-assisted. For larger areas, I often prefer to use ultrasonic-assisted liposuction in combination with the well-proven tumescent anesthesia method.

Is Liposuction Right for You? Questions to Ask Yourself

Have you made a real effort to lose weight?

Are you back to within 20 percent of your ideal body weight?

Do you have type 2 diabetes? Are you a smoker? Both can limit your wound-healing ability.

Are your love handles and other stubborn fat deposits really upsetting you?

Do you have realistic expectations? Liposuction can only remove small amounts of fat in selected areas. It isn't weight loss surgery.

Will you continue to eat well and exercise after the liposuction? Weight gain will undo the liposuction benefits.

Have you had previous abdominal surgeries or radiation treatment that produced scar tissue that could complicate the procedure?

In general, liposuction is a very safe procedure that can restore or reshape your body contours. Liposuction is right for you if you've been eating well, working out, and are back to or close to your pre-baby weight but still have bumpy areas that just won't go away. If you are planning a tummy tuck as part of your Mommy Makeover, this is an excellent time to do the lipo as well—you're already under anesthesia and planning some recovery time. If you are healthy enough and desire a bit more definition, liposuction can easily be added to a Mommy Makeover. Liposuction won't add much to your discomfort or slow down your healing greatly. If you choose liposuction alone, the recovery time is somewhat shorter than for the tummy tuck. Likewise, if you're planning a breast lift and augmentation, now's the time to also get rid of those little bra strap bulges. If you had a C-section, you might have a little bulge of fat just above the scar. Liposuction can take care of that too.

THE LIPOSUCTION PROCEDURE

Liposuction is performed with tumescent anesthesia with or without general anesthesia—many Mommy Makeover patients combine liposuction with their other procedures, so a general anesthetic is helpful here.

I begin the procedure by using a thin, straw-like stainless steel tube called a cannula to inject the tumescent anesthesia—a mixture of a local anesthetic (the numbing medicine), a blood constrictor, and normal saline solution (sterile salt water)—into the areas to be reduced. This makes the fat walls swell up and makes them easier and less painful to remove. If needed, I'll next use an ultrasonic tip on the cannula to help break down the fat. The high-frequency sound waves make the tissue near the tip vibrate very rapidly, which helps break down the connections between the fat cells and makes them easier to suck away. Next, I'll move the cannula carefully around in a fan shape within the area to be treated to make sure the fat is removed evenly. As I move the cannula with one hand, I'll be feeling the area with the other to make sure I don't leave any bumps, ridges, or depressions in the skin when I suction out the combined fluid and fat cells.

If you are also having a tummy tuck, I can insert the cannula into part of the area to be treated from the tuck incision. That means fewer scars. If you do end up with lipo scars because I couldn't reach everything through the original incisions, they are very small—just little puncture marks no wider than your fingertip. I can often hide the scars in an existing skin crease. They heal up very quickly, and because I have placed an anesthetic directly into the lipo area, you have very little pain for many hours afterward. If your liposuction is in addition to your tummy tuck, it really won't add to your post-op pain much at all.

Liposuction is quick. The longest part of the surgery is waiting for the tumescent anesthesia to take effect. When combining liposuction with other surgeries, we can inject the tumescent fluid and work elsewhere while it sets up. With a combination of skill and efficiency, liposuction typically adds no more than an hour to your Mommy Makeover surgical time.

AFTER LIPOSUCTION

After a brief stay in the recovery area, liposuction patients generally go home. You'll notice right away the areas that had liposuction may look worse now than they did before the procedure. That's because they're swollen from all the fluid I injected and from the effects of the surgery. The swelling and bruising will go down, but it will take several weeks or even longer for you to see improvement; it might be up to three to six months before the final result can be appreciated.

You'll be sent home wearing a tight-fitting, corset-like surgical garment to help with the swelling. Other than that, the postoperative instructions are pretty minimal. If you've also had a tummy tuck, you'll follow the post-op instructions for that. We definitely see the best results when you can wear the garment nearly all the time for six weeks. Some of my patients tell me that wearing it is actually more comfortable than not wearing it because it gives them a sense of security as they heal—like a long, gentle hug.

If you had liposuction alone, you won't have much pain, just some soreness that will go away in a few days. I'll prescribe a mild pain-killer to help alleviate that. Most of my patients don't need anything strong and stop taking even the mild meds after just a few days.

Liposuction is a very safe procedure, but there is always a very small chance of infection. As always, having type 2 diabetes or being a smoker could slow healing. The biggest complication of this surgery is contour irregularities. If too much fat is suctioned out of one particular spot, it can leave a depression in that area. When looking at the area as a whole, it can look a little wavy or show as "peaks and valleys" in your skin. In my experience, I have found that I can minimize or avoid this issue altogether by using my opposite hand as a "feeling guide" while performing the surgery.

Simply because of injected fluids working their way out, you might ooze a bit from your incisions the first night or two home after the surgery. Your body will have to absorb that fluid or push it out through the small incision holes. This fluid will sometimes be a light reddish color; that doesn't mean you're bleeding. As you begin to increase activity, even more fluid may appear. You shouldn't be alarmed by this. It's perfectly normal.

You can take a shower on your second day home (and it'll feel good!). Most of my patients begin to return to their normal activities within just a few days. Almost all are back to their usual activity level within two weeks.

You will visit me in my office within a week after the surgery to make sure you're healing well and again in a month or so for a quick checkup and review of your progress. I will see you again after three more months just to ensure all is healing well.

A strong word of caution: If you gain weight over time, you can still put fat back into the area we worked on or develop bulges in areas nearby. To keep the best results from your liposuction surgery, try to maintain your normal weight and avoid big weight gains and losses.

FURTHER POSSIBILITIES

Sometimes the fat I remove during the liposuction procedure can be processed and re-injected into your body to help fill out areas that are wrinkled or a little too flat. Fat is transferred commonly to the face, breast, buttocks, or hands. For wrinkles in the face, a small amount can be used to fill these in. Lips can be augmented with fat as well. Many times after breast reconstruction, since the skin remaining after the breast removal surgery is so thin, fat transfer can be performed to even out some of the contours. If you wish and it's appropriate, I can even transfer some of your own fat into your buttocks to help fill out the area and give it a bit of a lift.

I can also transfer fat into the backs of the hands. Because we naturally lose fat from this area as we grow older, this is a place where a mom can really show her age. Transferring fat can rejuvenate the hands, fill in wrinkles, and give them a more youthful appearance—

the improvement is often dramatic. The procedure is simple and fairly painless. You can expect some swelling and stiffness in your hands for a couple of weeks, but after that, you'll be back to your normal activities. And the improvement is *permanent*.

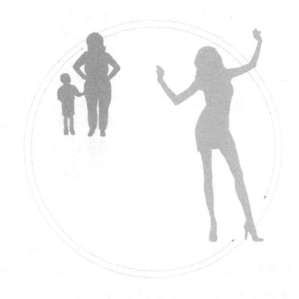

Chapter 15

BREAST PROCEDURES

She showed up for her 10 a.m. appointment at my office with a smile on her face, attempting to exude the confidence she had once felt. She said she had three kids, the youngest only a year old. She had breast-fed her until she was ten months old, same with the older kids.

"No," she said. She never really loved her breasts and had sometimes fantasized even before having babies about how she might improve them.

"And now?" I asked.

And then came the tears. With eyes in her lap, she described the changes.

"They're worse! The little that I used to have is all but gone! They're totally deflated up top, the nipples are on the floor, and I have to roll them up to fit them into a bra!" And then, wiping her tears, trying to smile again, she finally looked up at me and said, "Please say you can help."

I smiled at her and began …

Pregnancy and breast-feeding have a major impact on a woman's breasts, with the age at the time of pregnancy, the duration of breast-feeding, and number of children, all being factors. I have heard lots of stories from patients who have tried various things to prevent and minimize these changes, all to no avail. While you're breast-feeding, there's really nothing you can do to prevent the eventual sagginess and deflation. It's almost inevitable. The skin stretches from the milk production and from the stimulation from the child—the pulling and tugging that is a normal part of breast-feeding. While a bra with good support is recommended and can be helpful, it can't prevent sagging completely. Gravity takes hold. Genetics affect it. And all the changes that are a normal part of pregnancy contribute.

Your breasts go through a lot of perfectly normal changes as they swell with pregnancy, increase even more with breast-feeding, and then almost magically deflate when you wean the baby. At first, you'll probably feel great relief in the reduced size and tenderness. But then reality sets in and you realize that these are not what you started with—and they're not coming back. They're much flatter on top and much droopier below. There might be red stretch marks. And generally after subsequent children, the changes are exaggerated. The skin and tissue have been permanently stretched and altered and just can't spring back to where they were before. Often, as they change, one breast ends up a bit larger than the other. The nipples may be permanently widened, and the areola, the colored circle around the nipple, may be stretched out of shape. And, of course, the stretch marks will still be there.

Patients whose breasts might have been very full and perky, even voluptuous, before the babies, now describe their breasts as "runny sunny-side up eggs that shift and slosh around when they move," "deflated udders," "sad little sacks," and "pancakes with sausage nipples." I had one patient who complained that her children "sucked the life outta them." And patients who never really loved their breasts anyway also begin to envision what might be possible.

When we meet in consultation, I like to gain an understanding of your perspective on your breasts. Let me give you an idea of how some of these discussions have gone:

How do you feel about your breasts?

- "I just want them to look like they used to."
- "I can't stand them."
- "I don't even recognize them anymore."
- "I hate them."

How do you feel about the size of your breasts?

- "They've disappeared."
- "They're two different sizes."
- "They're too large and droopy."
- "They look awful."

How would you describe your breasts?

- "I no longer have any cleavage."
- "Saggy" or "droopy."
- "One is way bigger than the other."
- "They point in opposite directions."
- "They're just ugly, and I want to hide them."

Where are your nipples pointing?

- "They've been staring at the floor for a long time."
- "They definitely need a lift."

Some women can simply talk about all this lightheartedly and openly. Others find this part of the discussion very difficult. We always find a way to communicate. Breasts are an important part of how a woman sees herself, so I really want to get inside *your* thought process, to understand what *you* want.

As you begin to examine this decision, the real question to consider is this: What is most important to *you* about your breasts? Do you want them to be fuller, or do you want to be perkier? These two aren't necessarily mutually exclusive. I will share my professional experience and thoughts on what is most appropriate for your body type, but what *you* want, *your* vision, counts most.

We will also discuss timing. I generally prefer to do breast procedures on women who are not planning more children. An additional pregnancy and breast-feeding will again swell the breasts and stretch the tissue and skin. However, unexpected pregnancies have been known to happen—there's no reason to panic. Fortunately, breast-feeding after a breast lift is usually not a problem. We are very careful not to damage the nipple and the tissue underneath it during the breast lift operation. Because the skin has already been tightened up by the breast lift, the extra stretching from the new baby weight doesn't cause very much new sagginess; the implant that is already in place usually takes care of any deflation.

Additionally, we will talk a lot about being conservative in your Mommy Makeover. Where breast work is concerned, I tell my moms, "You probably want to be noticed as the mom of Jennifer and Jim and not because you are the mom of Jennifer and Jimmy with *those*." Moms at this stage in their life tend to be conservative anyway; you don't want people so busy looking at your chest that they miss who you really are and what is really important to you. On the other hand, you want to look your best at the kids' school functions and sports. And you want to feel and look fabulous to your partner and to others when you put on a nice evening gown and fill it out perfectly.

When my patients discuss the idea of having breast work done with their partners, a few issues usually come up. Most of them are the basic concerns about plastic surgery that we discussed in Part 1. The main issue related directly to breast procedures is size. Husbands are usually focused more on that issue and encourage their wives to go up in size. Initially, a husband and wife agree on cup size only about half of the time. I can help them work that out by using photographs, as well as a specialized sizing system, so they can get the idea of what the various sizes will look like.

The decision to have plastic surgery on your breasts gives you a chance to envision yourself as you always wanted to be. It's a chance to restore your appearance to match your age and also to help out where nature may have left you a little wanting.

IS BREAST SURGERY RIGHT FOR YOU?

There are several types of breast procedures for you to consider.

- Breast augmentation
- Breast lift (known as mastopexy)
- Combined breast lift with augmentation
- Breast reduction
- Nipple reduction/Areolar reduction/Nipple inversion correction

We will discuss all of these when we meet for our consultation. When you choose more than one, I usually recommend that we do them at the same time. It's faster, easier, and less expensive to do the procedures at the same time. The time in surgery isn't usually much longer, and the recovery period is the same.

Are You Ready for Breast Surgery?
Questions to Ask Yourself

How long has it been since you stopped breast-feeding? Your breasts take three to six months after you stop breast-feeding to take on their new and permanent form.

Are you planning on having any more children? If so, you may want to wait, as this might alter your result.

Do you want perkiness, or do you want fullness? How do you feel about your breasts? What would your ideal breasts look like?

Are you back to (or close to) your pre-pregnancy weight?

Is your overall health good? Breast work as part of a Mommy Makeover is very safe, especially in women who are relatively young and healthy.

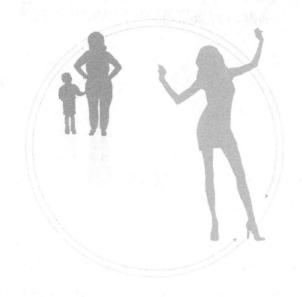

Chapter 16

BREAST AUGMENTATION

P regnancy and breast-feeding can certainly change the shape and size of your breasts. When you have weaned the baby and the swelling finally goes down, the upper part of your breast (what we surgeons call the upper pole) is likely to be flattened. The curvature and cleavage that once were there are now altered—or gone. The good news is that if you were dissatisfied with the size and shape of your breasts even before the baby, your Mommy Makeover can give you the breasts you have always wanted. In breast augmentation surgery, we insert an implant under each of your breasts to restore them to their earlier pre-pregnancy shape, size, and symmetry—or to reinvent them!

WHAT CHANGES DO YOU WANT TO SEE?

Our consultation will begin with questions like, "What cup size are you now?" and "Where do you desire to be?" Your augmentation will be designed individually for you and your body. Because of variations in body type, height, weight, and your vision for yourself, your implant size is a very specific personal choice. And, of course, this may be different from your friends who have had augmentations. Not all bodies are created equal—or even alike.

Cup size can vary from one bra manufacturer to another and one lingerie store to another. For that reason, I never guarantee a certain cup size postoperatively. But we will use cup size as a jumping-off point to start our conversation and then move on to some other important considerations.

If you desire a specific cup size, I will show you pictures and drawings to help you visualize the amount of fullness that is *possible* for you and will *feel* right to you. A lot depends on how much fullness you want on top. Sometimes, the larger the implant, the fuller you will be. Other times, we achieve fullness with a small base diameter that projects most of the substance forward, so you can actually be fuller without the larger implant. I will also work with you to visualize what your cleavage would look like with implants of various sizes. You'll be able to handle the implants, see how they feel, tuck them under your bra, and use a sizing kit so that you can "wear them" and see how they look. I will use specialized measurements, assess your skin stretch, and note your desired cup size. My well-defined process gives you a really good idea of how you're going to look after the surgery.

TYPES OF IMPLANTS

Breast augmentation implants fall into two basic categories. The first is the saline implant. This has a silicone shell, sort of like a rubbery balloon, that we fill with sterile salt water (saline) to the level of fullness you want. The other category is the gel implant. There are two different forms of gel implants; cohesive and form-stable gels. They are both made from a silicone shell like the saline implants, but they're each filled with a different type of medical-grade silicone gel. Cohesive gels have been improved recently with a thicker consistency than in the past and stay together better if there is a rupture. The makeup of the form-stable type is even thicker. They're nicknamed "gummy bears" because their consistency is very much like that of the candy. When you squeeze the form-stable gel, it bulges out a little bit, but when you release the pressure, it springs back to its normal shape. The "gummy bears" are initially a bit firmer than the cohesive gel implants, but they soften with time inside the body.

When women give the saline and gel implants the "feel test," the vast majority say, "The saline feels like a water balloon, and the gel feels more natural." Which is right for you? That depends. The saline implant is often used for the super-augmented look. They are less expensive but have a higher risk of problems (rupture, rippling, looking too fake, and a tight scar around the implant known as a capsular contracture). The gels look and feel more natural, resist the rippling, and last longer, with less risk of complications overall.

I often prefer to use the form-stable "gummy bears" for several reasons. Form-stable gel implants are anatomically shaped like a teardrop, which is maintained no matter your position (standing, lying, or doing headstands) and have a better resemblance to a normal, natural-looking breast. Due to the consistency of the gel, these tend to create the shape of the breast as opposed to taking on the shape of the existing breast, as the round gels do. When we insert these implants, most of the substance is directly behind and underneath the nipple, creating a larger, fuller result. The "gummy bears" also work very well for the patient who is very thin, without much natural breast tissue.

Having said all that, let me assure you that I do use all types of implants and know them intimately. This is a detailed discussion we will have when you visit my office so that you will feel well informed, educated, and comfortable with your choice for your specific needs and desires.

WHAT SIZE AND SHAPE?

Implants come in all sizes and shapes. This is also a very individual decision, one we will discuss in great detail. It all comes down to what you personally want your breasts to look like.

We will begin by matching the base diameter of the implant to *your* weight and body type. We will look at how wide the implant is when it is placed in position and how much it projects to the sides. If it is too large to fit inside the frame of your chest, it will sit in your armpit and make you look heavy. In this case, you may also be able to *feel* the edges, an unnatural and uncomfortable feeling. For a perky look, you want the implants facing straight ahead, not out in the armpit. Choosing the correct size implant will allow it to fit within your breast and give a natural appearance.

That brings up the matter of how much input does the spouse have? The old adage is that the husbands always want to go bigger on breast size. Today, that's not so true. A lot of the spouses are very supportive and want a size that's going to give the most comfort and confidence. We have you try on a sizing system to determine what size feels comfortable to you. Do some women rely on their spouse's input? Absolutely, but I still push the patient to tell me how *she* feels. Many times, I can tell her comfort level by some nonverbal cues.

So are you ready for the *ultimate dressing room* experience? This is the most exciting part of the consultation—when Mommy realizes that her dreams can actually become reality. This is the point where you really *see yourself* with a different chest size. And it is fun for all of us to get to see the excitement as the possibilities occur to you. "Oh! This is what I could look like! This is becoming more and more real. I can't wait!"

I use the Goldilocks approach to sizing implants. We try on too small and too large until we get it "just right." It is interesting how close (or how far off) patients can be in their original thinking about their perfect size. It is pretty easy to judge reactions once I get you in front of a floor-length mirror and you actually *see* the results staring back at you. By taking some time to listen and watch here, it is very rare that we fail to find just the perfect size for you. We do this together in the office so that I don't have to guess (or rely on an overzealous husband's input) in the operating room, when you're asleep. Gathering the above information, along with your reaction to the experience of trying on the sizing system, I will guide you in the choice of size, shape, and the style of implant I think is best for you and will give you the most confidence. To me, there's nothing sexier than confidence, and I think a lot of partners feel that way, too.

ARE BREAST IMPLANTS SAFE?

The most common question I get asked about breast implants is, "Are they safe?"

They are.

The earlier generation of implants had some problems and were subsequently reformulated. There were many questions of whether implants caused connective tissue or autoimmune diseases or worsened them. No cause and effect relationship was ever scientifically proven between breast implants and these diseases.

The silicone gels were returned to the market around 2009 after extensive research, testing, and reformulation were completed. They are now much stronger and less likely to rupture or ripple than the saline implants. The form-stable implants ("gummy bears") are even safer with the least chance of problems related to the implant.

THE BREAST AUGMENTATION PROCEDURE

A number of decisions have to be made regarding your breast augmentation. Here is an overview of what that entails.

Implant Placement

The first and most crucial step in the procedure is creating the pockets within the breasts to hold the implants. Pocket creation may involve manipulation of the pectoral muscles, which run from your shoulders down toward your belly button. If you put your right hand over your left breast, as if you were saying the Pledge of Allegiance, you're pretty much on top of your pectoral muscle on that side.

There are several ways to go about this:

- *Subglandular.* Above the pectoral (chest) muscles—The implant fits between the breast tissue and the underlying muscle.
- *Submuscular.* The implant fits completely underneath the pectoral muscle.
- *Dual plane* (partial submuscular). The implant fits behind the breast tissue and partly underneath the muscle.

Which location is best? In general (though I consider every surgery individually), I prefer the submuscular approach whenever possible. This location allows me to hide the upper aspect of the implant a bit under the muscle and gives a more natural-looking breast, with little to no rippling effect. It also allows for better mammograms because less breast tissue is distorted by the implant, and more of the breast can be accurately evaluated than if the subglandular approach is used. In Mommy Makeovers, I often use the dual plane position to achieve a bit of elevation for moms who want more fullness up top but don't quite need a full breast lift yet.

Incision Location

To reach the pectoral muscles, I will typically perform an inframammary incision, which goes under the breast within the inframammary fold, the natural crease where your breasts meet your chest. This incision is rarely longer than an inch or two. This approach allows me to place the implant very precisely and quickly, with minimal bleeding, and the scarring fades quickly, usually within a few months.

Other locations to place the incision include the transaxillary incision (where your breast meets your chest wall at the armpit), a periareolar incision (around the nipple), and a TUBA—a transumbilical breast augmentation. That's done through your belly button and can only be done using a saline implant. I rely on these approaches very rarely and will discuss them with you if they seem likely in your case.

Pocket location and the amount of dissection performed is key to obtaining excellent results with breast augmentation. If the pocket is aggressively overdissected, the implant has the opportunity to move, rotate, and end up in a less desirable location. This can also happen if an overly large implant has put excessive pressure and stretched out the tissue. I have seen patients after another surgeon has performed their augmentation complain of having a "side boob," as the implant now resides more in the armpit than on top of their chest—not pretty.

First Impressions

The implant surgery is quick, usually 35 to 45 minutes. You may initially, upon waking, be startled by your new breasts. As the swelling goes down over the next two to four weeks, the feeling that they are sitting too high (like you could rest your chin on them), or the fear that they are bigger than expected, will all be alleviated as your breasts settle in and begin to look like you had hoped. You will also adjust to the new perkiness of your breasts after having spent so much time dealing with their deflation from pregnancy and breast-feeding.

We work ahead of time to prepare you (and your family) for the roller coaster of emotions you are likely to experience. While at first you could think they are too big or too high, you may then move to thinking they are too small. This is a common initial response, which we anticipate and expect. I always advise my patients to allow time to get used to the new you. Usually after this process is completed, my patients tell me, "They're perfect, exactly what I wanted."

AFTER THE SURGERY

You will go home the same day of your surgery. Some patients need pain medication for a few days to deal with the minor discomfort from muscle elevation and implantation; many don't really need much. After the surgery, you'll wear a sports bra and can shower on day two or three. The incision is small and is covered with a small bandage. I like to perform this surgery on Thursday or Friday so that you will have the weekend to recover and be right back to work on Monday.

Plan to rest and just zone out for the first couple of days. By day three, I'll ask you to do some gentle range of motion stretches to help the muscles get used to being in a new position with the implants there. And, please, no heavy lifting at all for several weeks.

I will see you within a week to check on your progress and teach you how to massage your breasts according to implant type. This will help soften the muscles up and allow the implants to settle into place. I will give you a silicone scar cream to help minimize scarring.

I will want to see you pretty frequently during the first year after your surgery to check how the implants are settling in, take pictures, and just generally make sure all is going well.

MAINTAINING YOUR RESULTS

A short list of changes could affect your results over time:

- Weight fluctuation after surgery.
- Pregnancy and breast-feeding.
- Genetics related to how much your skin elasticity diminishes over time.
- Size of the implant—the bigger the implant, the more strain it will create on the skin and breast tissue over time.

POSSIBLE COMPLICATIONS

Breast augmentation surgery is very safe. As with all medical procedures, there can be some complications. I will list a few of them here, but, remember, they are rare—and we are equipped to deal with them should they appear.

- *Capsular contracture*—Your body forms a scar tissue lining around the implant (this is natural with any new substance we introduce into the body). When this lining shrinks more than normal during the healing, it can cause the implant to feel hard and unmoving and change the appearance of the breast. We guard against this with the type of incision and the type of implants we use.
- *Rupture*—If you were to have a car accident, take a nasty fall heavily on your chest, or develop a contracture, you could have a rupture. This is very easy to detect with saline, because you look obviously asymmetric, kind of like having a flat tire. If a rupture occurs with the newer generation gel implants, the gel maintains its

shape so well that it might not even be noticed. With saline implants, the longer it's in place, the greater the likelihood of rupture.

- *Rippling*—Typically, rippling is detected on the sides and underneath the breast. It's most commonly seen in very thin individuals with saline implants, rarely in round gels, and almost nonexistent in the form-stable implants.

Again, this section is not to scare you. Breast augmentation surgery is very safe. It is a quick outpatient operation performed on healthy individuals without much physiological impact on your body. And the results are immediately gratifying.

MAMMOGRAMS AND BREAST IMPLANTS

If you have breast implants, you should continue your regular schedule for mammograms. The implants can hide some of the breast tissue from view, so the Eklund view, a technique that pushes the implant back against the chest wall and pulls the breast tissue forward and around it, is used. It sounds uncomfortable but is really no different than the usual mild mammogram discomfort.

EFFECTS OF IMPLANTS ON MOM

One of the best parts of my job is watching how patients respond to their augmentations. Let me share a story about a patient of mine, Danielle.

Danielle came in a shy, quiet girl who was so unassuming you could hardly notice when she was in the room. Talking with her about her desires was a challenge, as she held her head down, hugged her chest in an attempt to make the embarrassing area disappear altogether, and spoke barely louder than a whisper. With her husband at her side, holding her hand, she told me her story: "I've always been embarrassed about my chest. Ever since middle school I hated changing in the locker rooms because of the huge difference I noticed between myself and all the other girls." With tears welling up in her eyes, she continued, "My mom used to try to take me shopping, but that only made matters worse. I could never find anything to fit, at least not in a way to make me feel feminine and attractive. When I look in the mirror at my chest, I feel like a boy." When I performed her exam, her embarrassment was palpable in the room. After the measurements and pictures were complete, she continued to try to hug herself into invisibility. During the *ultimate dressing room* part of the exam, with each successive implant size she tried on, she emerged slightly more from her withdrawn shell. When we got to the point of desired fullness, I could tell she was in for some significant changes in her life. I even saw the briefest of smiles at her reflection in the mirror that day.

As expected, the surgery went well; she healed perfectly. When she came in for her first postoperative visit, I almost didn't recognize her. She was proud, confident, looked me in the eye when we spoke, and couldn't stop beaming: "I haven't stopped looking at myself in the mirror! I can't believe they're mine! They feel so real!" After the exam, she asked if I could take some pictures, even though it was very early in the healing process. As we walked to the photo room, I had to gently remind her to close up her gown so she wouldn't expose herself to the office. "Oh, honey," she told me in her sweet Nashville accent,

"I've already shown them to just about everyone I know! What's a few more people?"

Another patient, Raquel, wanted to give the gift of breast augmentation to her husband for their twelfth anniversary. After two children she felt a bit deflated but not enough to need a lift. "I just want to feel pretty again," she told me during our interview. And she was worried that she didn't look as good as she used to for her husband. "I think this will give our marriage a spark, too," she told me. "That's why I want to do it for our anniversary."

After her successful surgery, she was thrilled with the results. When I inquired about her husband's reaction to her changes, she replied, "Oh, I've haven't let him touch them yet. He's like a starved cheetah in a cage with a bunch of wild antelopes. He's going crazy, and I love it!"

During her next visit, I inquired again about her husband's response. She told me simply, "He's very proud of you! And so am I! I love them!"

That's the type of profound result I love to see with breast augmentation surgery.

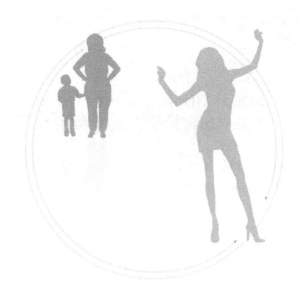

Chapter 17

BREAST LIFTS

O f all the sacrifices moms make for their kids, sagging breasts are one of the most visible. The swelling that occurs during pregnancy and breast-feeding cause the breasts to deflate and lose their elasticity—their lift. They become droopy and just flop on the chest. Many of my Mommy Makeover patients tell me that they want to restore their breasts to their pre-children form because they look so sad. I want them to be happy again.

Sagging breasts can be surgically restored with a mastopexy (a breast lift). We can raise and tighten the breasts, giving them back their lift. We can improve shape and symmetry, reposition the nipples, restore the effects of pregnancy and breast-feeding, and make them—and you—smile!

Breast Lift Readiness Quiz: What Changes Do You Want to See?

I start our discussions by asking you some questions to determine your vision:

What did your breasts look like before kids?

Were you happy with them?

Did you like your size?

Is there anything you always wanted to change?

Would you like your breasts to be perkier?

Do you want more fullness or size?

Some moms have always wanted larger breasts; some just want them back up in their original position; some want their nipples not to point to the floor. Some women actually loved the fullness, the increased cleavage, of their breasts while they were pregnant and want them to look like that now.

One of our goals for you is to have congruent breasts that have a natural appearance and shape. We can discuss the advantages of coupling the lift with an augmentation, not just for size but for symmetry, uniformity, and the overall look of the breasts when we are done. We want to avoid what is known as "Snoopy dog deformity," where an implant alone is used in an attempt to achieve a full lift.

There is a disconnect between the fullness created by the implant and the rest of the drooping breast—the nipple is the dog's nose pointing down. By lifting the breast tissue up on top of an implant, we can achieve a nicer cascade to the breast that has a natural-looking effect.

Another way of saying this is that pregnancy and breast-feeding flatten out the upper aspect of the breast. Also, doing a breast lift usually involves removing some tissue from the lower aspect of the breast. Augmentation compensates for these losses of volume and rounds out the result nicely. Using my advanced surgical techniques, I can perform both procedures at the same time, very safely. For these reasons, almost all of my Mommy Makeover patients decide on an augmentation with their breast lift.

BREAST-FEEDING AFTER A BREAST LIFT

As we discussed earlier, you can most likely breast-feed after a breast lift. When we do a breast lift, we do cut through some milk ducts; however, most of them will reform after several years. It is possible that if you do breast-feed after a breast lift, you may develop little pockets of trapped milk in your breasts. It won't affect the baby, but it can be a bit disconcerting to feel these temporary lumps until your body reabsorbs them. Because you may have short-term trouble with breast-feeding, and because pregnancy and breast-feeding may stretch out your breasts all over again, it might be best to wait until your childbearing years are over before doing the surgery. On the other hand, many of my patients want to enjoy the results from a breast lift earlier rather than later and choose to address the possibility for a little touch-up in the future, if needed.

BREAST LIFT EVALUATION

Breast lift surgery is generally very safe but not if you're a smoker. During the surgery, it is critical to maintain good blood flow to the nipple area. If you smoke, the nicotine makes all the tiny blood vessels in your body contract—in your fingers, your toes, and your nipples. I simply won't operate on anyone who hasn't agreed to abstain from smoking for six weeks before surgery to six weeks after. This is what I tell my smoking patients: "Every time you want to light up that cigarette, I want you to look down at your nipples and imagine them turning black and falling off." You must not have any nicotine at all, not even a nicotine patch or an e-cigarette.

I will also need to know if you have type 2 diabetes or high blood pressure. These conditions can also cause problems with blood flow to the nipple and can slow down incision healing. If these issues have been addressed and are under control, I can safely operate.

The first thing to examine is where your nipples currently reside. When your breasts are restored, the nipples should be back at the level of the inframammary fold (the point where your breasts meet your chest wall). Usually after a couple of pregnancies and breast-feeding, the substance of the breast and the nipple are lower (sometimes a lot lower) than the inframammary fold. We grade this ptosis (droopiness) on a scale. One is normal—your nipples are pointing straight ahead. Two is you're a little below the fold. Three is you're facing south. That helps me determine how much tightening you need and which surgical technique will be best.

BREAST LIFT PROCEDURE

This complex surgery involves excess skin removal, breast tissue shaping, and elevation of the NAC (nipple areolar complex) while maintaining blood flow to this area. It is important to note that the nipple is not taken off and put back on in a higher location, but a complete breast reshaping is performed.

The most common full breast lift procedure is known as the *Wise*, the *anchor pattern*, or *inverted T pattern*, because of the shape of the scar. This approach requires three incisions: one in a circle around the areola (used for nipple elevation and almost not visible due to the expected color changes between here and your breast), another going vertically down from the bottom of your nipple to the inframammary fold (which is the only really visible scar that fades quickly), and a third across the inframammary fold (which is mostly hidden beneath the breast). These last two let us remove excess tissue and skin to tighten up the breast. I have noticed in my patients that, about a year after surgery, I can barely see this scar from five feet away. Even if you are a swimsuit model and you wear a scanty bikini, the scar is usually hidden by the top.

In order to achieve total breast rejuvenation with skin tightening and improved fullness, an implant is often added to the lifting operation. In the past, many surgeons feared, and some still do, that this combined surgery would compromise the blood flow to the nipple. I have figured out a way that makes sense anatomically to maintain healthy blood flow while adding the implant in a minimally invasive manner. For many years, I have performed this combined breast lift-augmentation surgery successfully. By performing a breast lift in this fashion, the addition of the implant does not compromise blood flow any further, the surgery is just as safe, and ideal results can be obtained.

Depending on the size of your breasts and how droopy they are, the surgery will take anywhere from two to four hours. If we do augmentation at the same time, it usually adds about 30 minutes to the procedure. In the pre-op area, I draw some markings on your breasts to guide me. "Measure twice, cut once," is my motto. Most women's breasts are naturally a bit asymmetric—one is often a little bit larger than the other. Your surgery can make your breasts match better and get your nipples to line up with one another. But as I tell my patients, "They're sisters, not twins."

AFTER THE SURGERY

After a short time in the recovery area, you can go home. You may wake up with some numbness in your nipples from the local anesthetic placed during surgery. However, due to the amount of manipulation performed with this procedure, sometimes the nerves may act strangely for some time (numbness, diminished, or heightened sensations)—usually up to three to six months. You may feel some zapping and tingling sensations in your breasts as the nerves repair themselves. Be patient. Give it time. Only in rare cases is the numbness permanent.

I will send you home wearing a compression bra or a sports bra with a front clasp. For the first two weeks, it must be worn continuously. And for two weeks after that, it should be worn for at least 12 hours a day. Once the sports bra period is past, you can switch over to a regular bra (no underwires, please).

Some doctors like to install drains in your breasts to take off the fluid that inevitably forms after surgery. I think the drains are annoying, uncomfortable, and not really needed. I do ask that you keep an eye on your breasts for the first few days to see if one breast is getting more swollen or painful than the other. If that happens, I want you to call me so we can rule out some excess bleeding.

There will be some pain around the incisions for the first few days; it is usually treated with some mild painkillers (and muscle relaxants if the augmentation was also performed). You will be able to shower two days after the surgery. Sometime around days three to five, you will be back to light activities. Within one to two weeks, you should be back to full activity.

During the first month, there will be some swelling resolution. By the second month, your new shape is becoming apparent. By the fourth month, the shape really softens and you get that nice, round fullness in the whole breast. It is a good idea to wait to buy clothes or lingerie until then.

I will want to see you back one week after the surgery to check on your progress and remove any remaining bandages. I will see you again in a few weeks and then every few months for a year.

YOUR BREAST LIFT OVER TIME

Your breast lift should look great for a long time. If you gain or lose a lot of weight, or if you get pregnant again, the skin and tissue may be stretched again. Otherwise your breasts will continue to look good for many years.

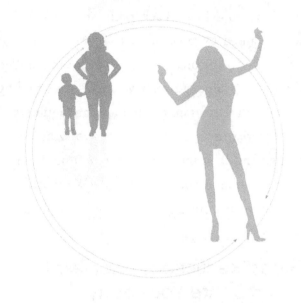

Chapter 18

BREAST REDUCTION

In some cases, breast reduction (reduction mammoplasty) is part of a Mommy Makeover. Large breasts will almost certainly get even bigger during pregnancy and breast-feeding. Though the breasts may regress a bit afterward, they can remain uncomfortably large. With mammoplasty, we can change the shape, reduce the size, and restore the symmetry of the breasts. We will also carefully reposition the nipples. Liposuction can be used to reduce the bulgy tissue around the bra strap area.

Aside from improving a mom's appearance, breast reduction can help quite a bit with the problems that sometimes accompany a very large chest. Upper and lower back pain, shoulder pain, and neck pain can all be caused by large breasts. There can be problems like rashes, chafing, and skin breakdown between and underneath the breasts. Women with large breasts have a hard time finding bras that fit; when they do, the bra straps can irritate the shoulders. Exercising, doing daily activities, even finding clothes to wear can be difficult and frustrating. And then there are the sometimes bold and unkind reactions of those around you to deal with. We know that reducing the breasts, even by just one cup size, can make a big difference.

Breast Reduction Readiness Quiz: Are You Ready?

What have you always wanted your breasts to look like?

What is your ideal cup size?

What does your partner think about smaller breasts? Is going down a cup size going to be a problem for him? (If so, we can discuss with him the practicality, the benefits, and the current impact on your life and your well-being.)

Did you stop breast-feeding at least six months ago? Your breasts need time to regress to normal before surgery.

Are you as close to your ideal weight as is realistic for you? Weight loss will show in your breasts as well as other parts of your body. However, women who are especially well-endowed cannot necessarily change their breast size by dieting.

Are you planning for more children? Although breast-feeding is perfectly possible after breast reduction surgery, temporary problems may develop.

Do you smoke? I will require that you stop smoking at least two months before the surgery and agree not to smoke for at least two months afterward.

Do you have realistic expectations about what can be done? The surgery can reduce your breasts by several cup sizes, but if your breasts are very large to begin with, they will likely still be a large size after surgery.

On the face of it, breast reduction surgery may sound like the opposite of what many moms want from their Mommy Makeover. However, a breast reduction isn't really much different from a breast lift; the breasts can be changed similarly in shape, symmetry, and nipple position. With a reduction, I'll just remove more breast tissue. But we need to be realistic about it. I have worked with women who range from F cups all the way to L cups. When the breasts are this large, sometimes the requests sound something like, "Just take them off. I want to be an A cup." Well, we can't really go from a very large cup all the way to an A—it is just too risky to remove that much tissue and maintain a viable nipple. Also, it might end up making a woman built to support much larger breasts look silly. Our goal is to achieve smaller breasts while keeping the breast size coherent to the rest of the body. And, because blood flow to the nipple has to be maintained through a certain amount of breast tissue, there is a limit to the amount of reduction we can do safely.

Cup sizes vary from store to store. Some stores go from A through DDD and then into the E, F, G, and H sizes. Some do DD, EE, and then FF. Once, a patient came in and told me that depending on the store her cup size was E, F, or G. My medical assistant was laughing because she thought I kept referring to this patient's breasts as *effing* Gs. I clarified, saying, "Yes, they were large, they were *either* Fs or Gs." We can usually reduce the breasts down to the DD or DDD range when they are that large.

Please understand that breast reduction is not weight loss surgery. Your breasts will certainly be smaller, and you'll be a bit lighter according to the scale, but the rest of your body will remain the same as before. As part of pre-surgery planning, I'll help you see how the surgery will change your profile. I'll show you how your breasts may drape over your belly because, after the surgery, your belly will be more exposed and may seem larger than before; it's just that you'll be able to see your belly better.

INSURANCE COVERAGE

Depending on how large your breasts are relative to your body weight and height and how much trouble you have experienced (and been treated for), you might be eligible to have your breast reduction surgery covered by your health insurance. There will certainly be a qualification process. This might include providing proof that:

- You have seen your primary care physician and/or your OB/GYN for this concern
- Different types (or numbers) of bras haven't helped provide the needed support when exercising or living your normal life
- You have explored alternative avenues: chiropractic, acupuncture, or physical therapy
- Your weight has been stable, and this is not being considered as a weight loss strategy

If and when your insurance company approves the procedure, they may try to dictate how many grams of breast tissue I need to remove for the procedure to be considered medically necessary. Understand that I will be making a professional decision about what is right for you, your body, and your desired results. I will consider how your breasts relate to your shoulders and your waist. I want your reduction to look appropriate for your body and to make a big improvement in your life. If it is a question of getting an aesthetically pleasing result or meeting a required weight, I will *always* stay with my own opinion to get the best result. If I think you are a borderline case for insurance approval, I will let you know up front. If that's the case, you can always elect to do this as a cosmetic procedure, paying for it yourself. We'll check your specific insurance benefits prior to scheduling surgery so you can make a decision that works best for you.

THE BREAST REDUCTION PROCEDURE

Procedurally, the basic breast reduction is very similar to the breast lift. This complex surgery involves excess skin removal, breast tissue shaping, tightening of the remaining skin to achieve elevation of the NAC (nipple areolar complex), and maintaining blood flow to this area. Here, however, we remove more tissue (sometimes as much as five pounds from each breast) and do more shaping.

We may use liposuction if you choose to have some of the fat around the bra straps removed; it is not often performed for a full reduction. We can also reduce the fat in the "tail" of the breast tissue where it meets the underarm tissue and the back. In some cases, we can extend the under-breast incision to the back and do something similar to a tummy tuck along the bra strap fold.

The reduction procedure takes about three hours, sometimes a little longer. Using liposuction or adding implants takes additional time. Larger breasts can be a bit more challenging and take a bit more time simply because they are bigger to work with. Almost all of my patients spend just a couple of hours in recovery and go home the same day.

AFTER THE SURGERY

After the surgery, you can expect some numbness in the nipples. This will fade over time (but could take as long as six months). The bigger your breasts, the greater the reduction, and the more likely the numbness will last for a few months. Be patient, and give it time. Almost everyone regains sensation within a year.

After the surgery, you will need to wear a compressive-type sports bra continuously for the first two weeks. After that, you can go to 12 hours a day for the next two weeks. Then you can go back to a regular bra (no underwires, please).

Because of the amount of tissue we remove in breast reduction, you may have some bruising in the area and some oozing from the incisions for the first few days. This is normal. Problems with wound healing and skin breakdown tend to be the most common complication. If you're overweight or have diabetes, the risk of wound-healing complications is much higher; upward of 50 percent of these patients will experience an opening in the wound. If you get one that opens up and oozes, we will treat it locally and give it time to heal from the inside out.

The pain after this procedure is generally quite manageable; we will prescribe some painkillers for the first few days. After that, you will likely be able to manage quite nicely without pain meds and switch to over-the-counter medication. Most patients are back to normal activities, except heavy lifting, within a week to ten days. The heavy lifting can be resumed around six weeks. You won't have any drains, and you will be able to shower after your second day at home. I will see you a week later to check on your healing. The scarring can be minimized by gentle massage and using a silicone scar cream.

During the healing, patients may sometimes develop masses in the breasts. These masses are not cancer. They are typically fatty necrosis—nodules that form in the area under and around the nipples because the blood flow isn't as robust as before. These masses usually soften and heal up on their own, but sometimes this necrosis can persist for longer than a year and might need to be removed. I require that my breast reduction patients get baseline mammograms before the surgery so we can determine that there are no preexisting issues. After the surgery, I ask you to check your breasts regularly. If you notice a lump, then you should consult with me before seeing any other doctor. I want to avoid you having a biopsy by a surgeon who doesn't realize that the blood flow has been altered. I want to prevent a false alarm cancer scare for you.

Your breast reduction should be trouble-free for many years. Fluctuations in weight can cause changes. You should try to maintain a stable weight (a good, healthy idea anyway). More importantly, though, the back pain, skin issues, and other problems caused by extremely large breasts will be *gone for good!* Some of my patients who came in all hunched over initially tell me, "I'm so much lighter up there that I feel like I'm falling backward!" These are some of my happiest patients (and it makes me smile, too) because I'm taking away their pain and making them look better.

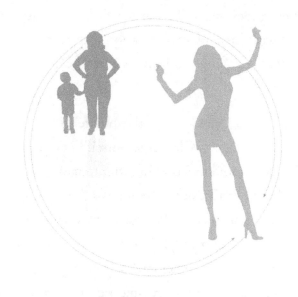

Chapter 19

OTHER BREAST PROCEDURES

A long with all the changes in mom's breasts that we have already discussed, there are a few others that arise with the areola and the nipples. These also can be corrected as part of your Mommy Makeover.

AREOLA REDUCTION

The areola is the circular, pigmented part of the breast surrounding the nipples. After breast-feeding, the areola may be widened or stretched past the point of no return. It may have become darker, larger, and even look puffy. This in itself can be unattractive, but if you have a breast lift and augmentation, the areola may seem disproportionately large afterward unless it is also reduced during the surgery.

Areola reduction doesn't affect the nipple, so it shouldn't affect your ability to breast-feed. The surgery itself is simple. I use a device that actually looks a lot like a cookie cutter to make a circular incision that is only skin deep all around the edge of the existing areola. Then I use a somewhat smaller cookie cutter to make another incision within the first (concentrically). I will remove the skin in between and sew the new edges together with dissolving sutures to make an areola that's smaller and more symmetric. The whole procedure is very quick—it usually only takes about ten minutes per breast.

Nearly all the areola reductions I do are part of other breast work in a Mommy Makeover. My patients generally don't experience any additional discomfort from the reduction as part of their breast lift. If you have only the areola reduction, the pain is minimal, and you can return to normal activities within a couple of days. The scarring is very minimal and fades to nearly invisible with a few months.

Most women heal up quickly from this procedure and end up with nice round areolas, but occasionally, the areolas will stretch a bit and become more oblong or oval. A lot depends on how much breast-feeding you did, how many kids you had, how much stretch is left in your skin, and how you heal. Healing may be a bit asymmetrical.

You may have some pigmentation changes during healing; sometimes the area will look a bit splotchy. But that usually goes away on its own. Some women experience loss of sensation in the area, but it almost always returns within six months. The improvement is permanent.

NIPPLE REDUCTION

After breast-feeding, a mom's nipples may not regress back to their normal size. Breast-feeding can cause the nipples to become permanently elongated, widened, and appear very stretched-out. They're either droopy and point south or seem to project out too far. Sometimes the nipples are asymmetrical, with one larger than the other. Enlarged nipples can make a mom feel very unattractive and self-conscious. They also make it hard to find a bra that fits comfortably.

Breast-feeding can definitely be affected by nipple reduction. It's still very possible to breast-feed, but there can be problems that would prevent it, so I typically ask my patients to delay this procedure until they are pretty sure they're done having kids.

Nipple reduction can be done as part of a more complete Mommy Makeover or on its own. As there are many different ways to perform this procedure, I will examine your body and individualize the treatment plan to you and your specifics.

My goal is to keep the blood flow to the nipple strong and to end up with a nipple that can still breast-feed and is still sensitive and responds to normal stimuli. Sensation in the area is often reduced at first, but the numbness gradually goes away. Because I almost always do nipple reductions as part of a Mommy Makeover, the very mild additional pain is just part of the bigger procedure. If you should desire only a nipple reduction, it can be done as an office procedure under local anesthetic, and you go home the same day. The pain of a nipple reduction alone is fairly minimal, and you can get back to your usual activities in just a couple of days. If there is any scarring at all (often there is none), it is very minimal.

INVERTED NIPPLES

I sometimes see patients with inverted nipples—the nipples are pulled inward instead of projecting outward. The inversion can be caused by breast-feeding or just by the sagging of droopy breasts. Because nipple inversion can also be a sign of breast cancer, the first thing I ask is that you see a family doctor to rule out this possibility. Once you have the go-ahead, we can proceed to discuss the solution.

Normal nipples are everted—they stand out naturally from the areola. The nipple is held erect by a cylindrical column of muscle. When that muscle column is damaged or just not very strong, the nipple inverts. Some women are simply born with this condition; it is caused by constrictions or adhesions in the milk ducts. Sometimes, breast-feeding will actually correct this condition, but sometimes it gets worse with attempts at breast-feeding and can actually be painful. Because of the scarring caused by the condition, the nipples might stay inverted, press on the milk ducts, and prevent breast-feeding.

Besides the concern of not being able to breast-feed, young women come to me because inverted nipples look unnatural and can make you feel self-conscious. They can also cause infections and rashes in the area.

To fix the problem, I elevate the nipples a bit and push them out of the breast. I use a tiny suture as a sort of hammock that I stitch into place under the nipple. It supports the base of the nipple so it everts outward and can't be retracted back in. Another approach is to take a little wedge of tissue from the base of the muscle cylinder and tuck that up underneath to provide a permanent support system.

Correcting inverted nipples is a fairly quick and simple procedure; it can be done under local anesthesia, generally takes only about 30 minutes, is not very painful, and leaves little to no scarring. You can generally resume normal activities within a day or two. If you want to try breast-feeding after the procedure, you will need to wait for the area to heal completely, usually a couple of weeks.

No matter which approach I use, I do everything I can to maintain blood flow and sensation to the nipple. I am also careful to preserve the milk ducts because I want you to be able to breast-feed if you wish. However, I cannot promise that outcome. I am also careful not to overcorrect the problem so you don't look like your nipples are permanently erect.

The goal, as with all breast surgery, is to restore your body and give you a pleasing and natural look.

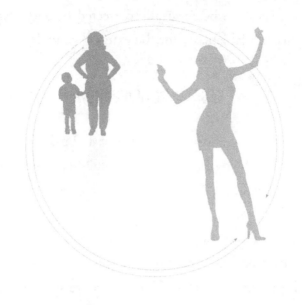

Chapter 20

LABIAPLASTY AND VAGINAL REJUVENATION

You're a mom, so you know that having a baby is like pushing a bowling ball out through a drinking straw. It's no surprise, then, that this has an effect on your vagina and external genital area. For some women, the vagina is stretched to the point where it makes intercourse unsatisfying. The labia minora (interior vaginal lips) and labia majora (external vaginal lips) can also end up stretched out, enlarged, and misshapen. Sometimes the clitoral hood is also enlarged.

All these issues can be surgically corrected through vaginoplasty for the vagina and labiaplasty for the external genitals.

VAGINAL REJUVENATION

After the vagina has been stretched by childbirth, it doesn't always return to its pre-baby tightness. The more children you have, the more your vagina is stretched. An overstretched vagina can keep you from having satisfying sexual function. The surgical fix for this is called vaginal rejuvenation or vaginoplasty. It is actually a simple operation that uses a stitch or two to help tighten the vaginal opening, making a tighter fit during intercourse. The procedure strengthens the area and restores the inner and outer muscles.

Because this is more a functional than a cosmetic procedure, both gynecologists and plastic surgeons can perform this procedure successfully. If, however, you desire a combination of the two procedures (vagina and labia), the vaginoplasty can be included in the labiaplasty surgery and should definitely be performed by an experienced plastic surgeon. A plastic surgeon, with his or her trained eye, will achieve aesthetically pleasing results in a way that a gynecologist usually cannot.

LABIAPLASTY

By itself or as part of your Mommy Makeover, I can correct any problems with the appearance of your external genitalia. Some women are hesitant to bring up the topic and are often embarrassed to discuss this with a male doctor. I understand the reluctance, but I encourage you not to feel that this or any other aspect of your body is something shameful or too personal to discuss with me. I want you to be happy with every part of your body and will help you discuss it comfortably. With today's trend of close grooming in the genital area, many women are very much aware of their appearance and want to do something about it. Labiaplasty (even for women who have never had children) has become much more popular in the past couple of decades.

Hormonal changes during pregnancy, combined with childbirth, can enlarge and stretch out the internal and external labia and the clitoral hood. The labia are now bigger and may also be uneven in size and shape. I want you to wait a minimum of three to six months before doing a labiaplasty so the swelling is resolved and the healing is complete. If you experienced any tears or trauma during childbirth, I want all to be back to normal before we even consider labiaplasty.

Many women start life with naturally asymmetric labia—they're just born that way, but childbirth can make the problem worse. The clitoral hood can become larger and thicker and covers more of the clitoris.

All this can make a mom feel very self-conscious about her intimate appearance. Enlarged labia can make intercourse physically uncomfortable and also cause discomfort when you're working out or wearing tight-fitting clothing (think swimsuit or skinny jeans). An enlarged clitoral hood can decrease sensation when having sex. Labiaplasty can decrease and alter the shape of the vaginal lips and help restore the area to a more youthful and attractive state.

Labiaplasty has three major components:

- Labia minora reduction
- Labia majora reduction
- Clitoral hood reduction

These procedures can be part of a Mommy Makeover or done separately (or individually) as outpatient surgery under local anesthetic with a blood constrictor to minimize pain and bleeding. The procedure, in any form, takes only about an hour.

To reduce and reshape the labia, I remove an asymmetric, wedge-shaped portion of the tissue and then suture the remaining tissue into a natural shape. I will not only reduce the size of the labia, I will make them more even and symmetric. I will also remove any excess tissue in the vaginal hood area.

I carefully orient the incisions so that scarring doesn't cause problems as the area heals. I don't want the vaginal opening to get tighter or to pull on the internal vaginal tissue. I use dissolving sutures to hold everything together. Most of the scarring will be invisible inside the vaginal tunnel. I hide the external incisions in the natural creases of the area; they usually fade away quickly anyway. If the clitoral hood is covered up, I can extend the incision or make a separate incision to expose the clitoris a bit more. While many women find this increases their enjoyment of sex, I am very careful not to remove too much in this area. Overstimulation can be more uncomfortable than enjoyable. And we need to ensure that the clitoris is still protected and doesn't get irritated.

AFTER THE SURGERY

Surgery in the genital area sounds like it ought to be really painful, but in fact, it's not too bad. Most of my patients who do it separately from their Mommy Makeover need very little pain medication and are back to their usual activities quickly. Because the area is much like the inside of your mouth, it heals quickly, just as a small cut inside your cheek does.

Once you are back home after the surgery, you will surely have some swelling, maybe some oozing, even a little bleeding in the area, especially during the first 24 hours. For several days following, there will be some soreness and irritation; we treat this successfully with mild painkillers and an ice pack.

We will send you home with a handheld squirt bottle (peri bottle)—you'll remember this from your postpartum self care. Simply fill the bottle up with an antibiotic solution, such as Betadine (povidone iodine) and rinse yourself after you urinate and when you are showering. Be very gentle at first. Use the bottle for about a week until the incisions are healed.

Labiaplasty is generally very, very safe. Infection, bleeding, and an overabundance of scar tissue are rare complications. Should you develop a hematoma (a bit of pooled blood) in the area, it could swell and be painful, but it isn't dangerous—and it's easy to treat, so please call me right away.

For the first month or so after the surgery, you will need to avoid using tampons; pads are fine. To avoid infection, skip baths, hot tubs, and swimming for three weeks. We do recommend sitz baths after each bowel movement during this healing period to ensure the area is cleaned well. And no intercourse for six to eight weeks until you are completely healed.

Your new appearance shouldn't change over time or even with more children. As always, it's a good idea to avoid excessive weight gain or loss.

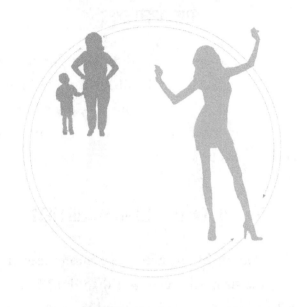

Chapter 21

FACIAL PROCEDURES

Years of sleepless nights during pregnancy and tending to young kids in the house can leave a mom with wrinkled, droopy eyelids, permanent bags under her eyes, and more wrinkles in her face than she would like. Your eyes make you look tired all the time (and you probably are!), but you don't need to look constantly exhausted or haggard. The good news is that, as part of your Mommy Makeover, we can address these issues and incorporate facial rejuvenation into your treatment regimen.

THE TIRED EYES

After all the sleep you've sacrificed for your family, now it's time for you. A blepharoplasty (an eyelid lift) will remove the droop and the bags and will help take years off your appearance. You can do this as part of a Mommy Makeover or as a separate procedure, perhaps along with other facial procedures.

DO YOU REALLY NEED AN EYELID LIFT?

Maybe not. You might just need to get more sleep (I know, as a father of four, that is much easier said than done). You might also have seasonal allergies that are giving you bags under your eyes. And sometimes, it's not the eyes that are the problem; it's the "elevens," those two vertical lines between your eyes, also known as frown lines or glabellar lines. They can give your eyes a tired appearance and can also make you look stern and unapproachable.

The appearance of frown lines can be quickly improved with injections of botulinum toxin. Botox is the more popular formulation of this toxin, but there are other drugs (Dysport and Xeomin) that work just as well. For ease of use, I'll use the word "Botox" to mean any of these three drugs. Botox is a toxin that temporarily paralyzes the muscles that form frown lines and keeps them from contracting. To relax frown lines, I will inject the Botox into five separate points between and over your eyebrows, using a fine needle that doesn't really hurt. Botox can typically be used between the eyes, on the forehead, and around the sides of the eyes (crow's feet). Occasionally, it can also be used for "smoker's lines" around the lips as well.

A caution here, though: If you are pregnant or breast-feeding, you must not use any form of botulinum toxin. The very small risk of the toxin spreading and affecting the baby is still too great to be considered acceptable.

If you prefer a more permanent fix, it's time to think about an eyebrow lift. The eyebrows might appear heavy because of the downward pull of the muscles between your eyes. A brow lift can fix this by selectively removing the muscles that pull the eyebrows down to form the "elevens." With these muscles gone, the forehead muscles take over and gently elevate the brows to a more appropriate height. I often combine the brow lift and the eyelid lift into the same surgery. Think of the eyebrows and eyelids working together like a curtain rod and a curtain. This combo surgery will help raise the curtain rod (the brows) as well as remove the bunching of the curtain (upper eyelids). Many times, if the eyebrows are not lifted at the same time, the effect of the eyelid lift is diminished. For more information on a brow lift, please visit our website www.musiccityplasticsurgery.com/browlift.

WHAT AN EYELID LIFT CAN DO

Eyelid surgery is very helpful in removing loose and sagging skin on the upper eyelid and loose skin and wrinkles on the lower eyelid. It's also great for reducing puffiness in the eyelids by removing the bulging fatty stores. The surgery also removes bags from under the eyes and restores the natural skin color there. In general, I aim to restore the natural contours of your eyes and give them a more rested and youthful appearance.

I cannot, however, change the basic shape and structure of your eyes and the area around them. As with all plastic surgery, it's important to have realistic goals and expectations.

Eyelid Lift Readiness Quiz

Has getting more sleep improved the appearance of your eyes? If not, or if the improvement isn't enough, a lift might be needed.

Do you have seasonal allergies that cause watery eyes, bags under the eyes, and other visible changes around your eyes? If your eyes look better when it's not allergy season, talk to your doctor about antihistamines. If your eyes still look unattractive when allergy season is over, think about an eyelid lift.

Do you drink alcohol often? You might have baggy eyes the next morning. Cut back on alcohol to see if this makes a noticeable difference.

Are you prepared to spend a couple of weeks with swollen eyes after surgery? Bruising and swelling might make you feel uncomfortable in a social setting for two to three weeks.

THE EYELID LIFT/BROW LIFT PROCEDURES

Eyelid lifts are typically done under general or local anesthesia or intravenous sedation. The surgery is very safe. If I do upper and lower lids only, the surgery takes about two hours. If we do a combo with the brow lift, it takes 30 to 60 minutes longer. And either way, you go home the same day. The recovery time is fairly short; any pain can be easily managed with mild medication.

To correct problems with the upper eyelid, I make an incision that runs along the natural crease of the eyelid. I use that space to remove fat pockets and excess skin and to tighten up the muscles. Because the incision is hidden in the crease and closed with very tiny sutures, the scar from it is basically invisible. For the lower eyelid, I make an incision just below the lower lash line where I can remove excess fat and skin and tighten up the muscles in the lower lid and in the bags underneath. I sometimes use a transconjunctival incision, which is made into the inner part of the bottom eyelid. The under-lash incision is closed with the same sutures; the scar quickly fades away to become nearly invisible.

AFTER THE SURGERY

You will be in recovery for a short time, during which I will remind you of possible complications. A small amount of swelling and bruising is normal. But if there is a lot of swelling or pain in one eye or any sort of change in your vision, it could mean bleeding into the eye socket, which could cause optic nerve compression. There are not many emergencies in plastic surgery—but this is one of them. Call me at once.

Though eyelid lifts are very safe, you may experience some slight bleeding just after the surgery. The risk of infection or other problems is very low; I will give you some antibiotic ointment to apply to the incisions twice a day for a few days. Pain from this procedure is usually not very severe and can be easily handled with mild painkillers. Just after the surgery, your eyes will likely be pretty swollen and bruised and may remain so for the next few weeks. The best treatment for the swelling is a lot of ice packs to the eyes. This is especially important during the first few days. Some patients have trouble closing their eyes at first; this is normal and changes quickly. As a precaution, I will prescribe ointment and drops to protect your eyes from getting too dry. The worst swelling will go down within a week to ten days. Once that happens, you can pretty much resume your normal activities, but no heavy lifting, please.

Until the swelling goes down, you probably won't be able to appreciate your rejuvenated eyes. Don't worry! You will soon look more energized and alert. It will take several weeks of anticipation before you see the full benefits of the surgery.

For the next six months, you should avoid exposing your incisions to direct sunlight. We want to protect the delicate skin of your eyelids as it heals. If you must be in the sun, wear big Hollywood-style sunglasses and a hat with a brim. After that, plan to maintain lifelong sun protection practices. Too much sunlight will age the skin and bring back the wrinkles. For most patients, the good results of an eyelid lift will last for somewhere between 10 and 20 years. The aging process continues, however, and gravity and your genes will always win in the end.

OTHER FACIAL REJUVENATIONS

Other facial rejuvenation procedures include filler or fat transfer to the cheeks, nasolabial folds (lines from nose to lips), marionette lines (from corner of mouth to chin), and lips. And, of course, the pinnacle of facial rejuvenation surgery, the facelift. Since this area of plastic surgery is advancing rapidly, I refer you to our website for the most updated information. Check out these pages:

www.musiccityplasticsurgery.com/non-surgical-facial-rejuvenation

www.musiccityplasticsurgery.com/facelift

www.musiccityplasticsurgery.com/juvederm-voluma-xc

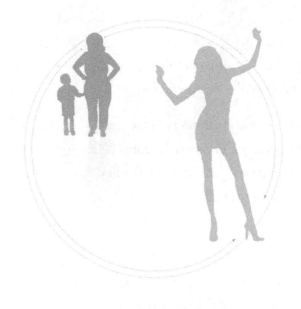

Chapter 22

SKIN CARE

To enhance their Mommy Makeover, many of my patients choose to add facial and skin-care products to their daily regimen. Since this is a time of childbearing age, I encourage them to use products that are safe during pregnancy and breast-feeding. Your skin is your largest organ, so anything you put on your skin can enter your bloodstream and could end up affecting your baby; it's imperative we choose products that are safe for you and your (potential) baby. This chapter is a description of our recommendations and the reasoning behind them.

In my practice, I have my patients work closely with my staff aestheticians, trained professionals in skin-care and beauty products. Beginning a healthy skin-care practice is a good start down the path of the Mommy Makeover; I encourage you to start early.

For many cosmetic products, there are no human studies to prove safety in pregnancy and breast-feeding. Because it just isn't ethical to ask women to participate in these studies, potentially putting their babies at risk, we don't have a lot of data to work with. There are animal studies, but they don't always translate into safety in human use.

So, at my office, we have one very firm rule about cosmetic products: *when in doubt, leave it out.*

Our skilled aestheticians will guide you toward products we know are proper for use during this important time in your and your baby's lives. Depending on your personal situation, there are a lot of areas to consider: routine skin care, sunscreen/sunblock, acne, stretch marks, hair products, Botox, lighteners, and growth factors. We will take these one at a time.

ROUTINE SKIN CARE

For all women, I recommend a facial cleansing routine that includes a cleanser, an exfoliator, and a moisturizer. I like plain Ivory soap. It's inexpensive, widely available, has no additives, and works really well.

A strong word of caution: For exfoliating during pregnancy, products with chemicals such as alpha hydroxy acids should be avoided. And during this time, you should stay away from chemical peels. Also avoid electrical stimulation (microcurrent) that affects collagen, as it can theoretically cause miscarriage; the risk is just not worth the benefit. Be careful not to use this even if you just think you might be pregnant. We also do not perform laser skin treatments on pregnant women because we do not have enough information on its safety or potential risk during pregnancy.

So you ask, "What can I do for exfoliation?" During pregnancy, skin brushing to remove dead cells from the surface of the skin is the only proven safe way to exfoliate. We recommend using an electric exfoliating brush with rotating heads. You can definitely use a manual brush. However, the rotating heads help penetrate deeper into the skin yet are still very gentle. It is quite easy to scrub without a lot of physical effort. The electric brush is portable and runs on a rechargeable battery. The result is superior to a manual brush.

SUN PROTECTION PRODUCTS

Ultraviolet (UV) radiation from the sun or tanning salons is the enemy of your skin. It causes wrinkles and dryness, and, during healing from surgery, prevents scars from fading well. The ultraviolet light in sunlight is in two forms: ultraviolet A (UVA) and ultraviolet B (UVB). UVA rays age your skin by breaking down the supporting fibers. UVB rays cause skin cancer. You would like to avoid both, but it is especially important to avoid the UVB light—it is more dangerous. Tanning booths use UVA light, which will definitely age your skin. I strongly suggest you avoid tanning salons at all times but especially while you are pregnant. Your skin is already stretched; don't damage it further. Also avoid the use of spray-on tanning products while you are pregnant because they contain dihydroxyacetone

(DHA). This ingredient gives your skin color, but your body may absorb between 1 to 15 percent of it. Remember that products you put on your skin can enter the bloodstream, so it can be like feeding it to your unborn baby.

Now let's talk about products that block UV light. They fall into two basic categories: sunscreens and sunblocks.

Sunscreens are lotions containing chemicals such as avobenzone and oxybenzone to filter out the UV rays. They are effective, especially the ones with high sun protection factors (SPF), but they wash off or sweat off easily. Regarding use during pregnancy, there are concerns that the chemicals may be absorbed into your system. Also, they are not as good at blocking UVB light as the sunblocks are.

Sunblocks are basically the same as the thick white ointments you used to see lifeguards using on their noses. They contain minerals, usually zinc oxide or titanium, to effectively block both UVA and UVB rays. In the newer formulations, the zinc or titanium is micronized so the particles are very small and not visible. Many cosmetic manufacturers put them in makeup now. The sunblocks tend to feel a little cake-like; they can plug up your pores and lead to acne. They are, however, unlikely to be absorbed into your body, so they are probably safe to use during pregnancy and breast-feeding.

And a word here about protecting all the parts of your body while out in the sun: A lot of women are careful about their face but forget about their chest, neck, décolletage area, and the backs of the hands. After the face, these are the most telltale areas to show sun damage and aging, but they are often neglected. When you're driving, for example, the backs of your hands are very exposed to UV light, even if it's cloudy outside. In addition to sunblock, be sure to wear large, dark sunglasses and a wide-brimmed hat—you want to protect the back of your neck, a most vulnerable spot. You need not go to extremes in covering yourself up; you should enjoy yourself outside! Some sun exposure on bare skin is actually beneficial so that your body can make enough vitamin D. Because of indoor jobs and concerns about sun damage, most of us don't get enough sunshine to make adequate vitamin D; consider talking to your doctor about a daily supplement if you feel you might be deficient.

ACNE PRODUCTS

Hormone changes during pregnancy and breast-feeding can cause acne (often mild, sometimes more severe). As annoying and unsightly as acne is, it is important to *be very careful* about treating it. Many standard acne solutions are not at all safe for you or your baby during this time. This can be a bit complex, so I have made a list below with my comments on each.

- *Topical treatments such as benzoyl peroxide.* We have conflicting information. Manufacturers say that only about 5 percent is absorbed into the skin, that what gets absorbed is completely metabolized, and that it shouldn't affect the baby. I think these products are probably safe but encourage you to consult your doctor before using them—and when in doubt, leave it out.
- *Prescription creams with antibiotics.* We don't have great studies to rule out the risk of systemic absorption and possible harm to the baby. When in doubt …
- *Products containing glycolic acid.* These have been studied in animals but not in humans. Although any systemic

absorption is probably minimal, if you have any concerns, leave it out.

- *Acne products with sulfur.* These may pose a risk to your unborn baby.
- *Topical products containing beta hydroxy acid (BHA) or salicylic acid.* These also fall into the not-studied-in pregnant-women category. Because you may absorb some of these products through your skin with unknown effect, *leave them out.* Also check the labels of all skin creams, not just acne products, for these chemicals.
- *Accutane (isotretinoin) and Retin-A (tretinoin).* There are stern warnings from doctors about the dangers of these products during pregnancy. These drugs have a *real* risk of causing congenital malformation (birth defects) and miscarriage. *Leave them out!* Stay away from any sort of retinoid treatment. That means tretinoin, isotretinoin, tazarotene, and adapalene, in any form, oral or topical, during pregnancy and breast-feeding.

So I can hear you saying, "What can I use for acne during pregnancy?" Glycolic acid and exfoliating scrubs are safe. Just don't overdo it. I like to simply encourage you to stay with the drug-free approach: gentle washing twice a day with Ivory soap, followed by a moisturizer. It's safest that way.

STRETCH MARKS

Stretch marks are caused by the expansion and stretching of the skin during pregnancy, most often in the breasts and the belly.

They are basically a mild form of a scar—and they're permanent. No magic creams, lotions, or special ointments will prevent them or remove them. Your tendency to develop them depends mostly on your genetics. If your mother got a lot of them, you likely will, too. It also depends on how rapidly you gain weight during pregnancy. The faster the weight gain, the more likely they are to appear. Hydration during pregnancy is the best defense. Drinking plenty of water will keep your skin elastic and better able to manage the stretching.

When you decide on a Mommy Makeover, I often end up removing some stretch marks with the skin that we remove during breast and tummy procedures.

HAIR PRODUCTS

I strongly recommend against hair dyes and coloring if you might get pregnant anytime soon or if you're breast-feeding. The dye chemicals that go on your hair can find their way into your body and harm your baby. Even "natural" dyes such as henna can be a problem. Just leave it out for now. And because we want to guard against any kind of harsh chemical during this important time, perms are out, too. I recommend you just go "au naturel" for now. Once you are done having babies and decide on your Mommy Makeover, you can change your hair color even as you give your body a more youthful appearance.

BOTOX

I discussed this in chapter 21, but it is important to emphasize it here again. Botox, Dysport, as well as fillers such as Restylane or

Juvederm need to be *avoided entirely* during pregnancy and breast-feeding. These are rated category C by the FDA, which means that we simply don't have enough information to know if these products are safe during pregnancy and breast-feeding. *Leave them out.*

LIGHTENING AGENTS

The lightening agent hydroquinone, also known as tocopherol, is often used to blend out age spots and pigmented areas. It has a high systemic absorption rate, ranging from 35 to 45 percent. *Leave it out* during pregnancy and breast-feeding.

GROWTH FACTORS

Growth factors, some of the latest advancements in skin care, are used in many products to help the body repair and renew collagen in order to correct signs of aging. These products may be quite remarkable in helping an aging mom's face, but they may be detrimental to a developing fetus. Again, there are not enough studies to make me comfortable in recommending their use during pregnancy and breast-feeding.

These are our recommendations in an attempt to maintain safety during this potential time of pregnancy and breast-feeding. As with any product, treatment, or even food, always check with your OB/GYN to ensure safety to you and your baby. And remember, when in doubt, the safe option is to *leave it out.*

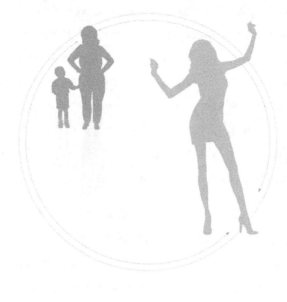

Chapter 23

HEALTHY EATING FOR MAINTAINING YOUR MOMMY MAKEOVER

You're a mom, so you've already learned a lot about what foods to eat and what foods to avoid during pregnancy and breast-feeding. The same foods you ate to ensure a healthy pregnancy will help you maintain the benefits of your Mommy Makeover. Eating well and drinking lots of plain water will help keep your skin elastic and avoid sagging and wrinkling. Also, you want to eat well to avoid weight swings—big gains and losses will stretch out and undo the tightening you achieved in your lift procedures and liposuction.

Any foods high in antioxidants will be very beneficial. They are easy to recognize since most are quite colorful. Blueberries and pomegranates are your friends because they contain anthocyanin, which helps protect your skin from fine lines and dryness. They also provide lots of vitamin C, which you need to produce collagen to keep your skin full and plump. In general, all colorful fruits and vegetables are high in antioxidants, which prevent the free radical damage that can be the precursor to fine lines and wrinkles that age your skin.

Orange vegetables, including sweet potatoes, carrots, and butternut squash, contain beta carotene, which your body converts to vitamin A and to retinol, which helps smooth the skin and protect it from sun damage. Spinach and kale are other great sources of beta carotene.

Dark chocolate—in moderation—is another great choice. It's full of antioxidants and flavonoids, which help with skin repair.

Walnuts, fish, avocados, flax seeds, tofu, soy milk, and edamame (soy beans) are all great sources of omega-3 fatty acids, which help provide smoother skin and healthier hair. The soy foods also contain isoflavones, which help reduce inflammation and can help stave off collagen breakdown to improve your skin tone and minimize wrinkles. Fish oil capsules are also a good source of omega-3s, but be cautious with these. They can thin the blood. Never use them in the third trimester of pregnancy. And if you are planning any sort of surgery, including a Mommy Makeover, stop taking them at least two weeks in advance.

Green tea is an excellent source of antioxidants, especially the kind called catechins. These can help prevent skin cancer and may help stave off damage from sunburn.

By sticking to a regular exercise regimen and incorporating these foods into your diet in moderation, you should be able to maintain your beauty and the results of your Mommy Makeover.

AFTERWORD

The Mommy Makeover in Action

Let me share the story of a Mommy Makeover patient who had amazing results.

The patient (I will call her Anne) was in her late 30s and had already delivered and breast-fed three healthy boys. That takes a toll on a mommy—in this case, especially her breasts. She was totally flattened on top and saggy on the bottom. She had, for some time, been thinking about a Mommy Makeover with breast lift and augmentation and a tummy tuck, but she had a busy family life, a demanding professional schedule, and a husband to consider. So she kept putting it off and having second thoughts about whether she really wanted to spend money on herself like that. How would she get the time away? Would the kids suffer? Would work be a problem? Should she spend that money?

Her husband (call him Joe) was very supportive and made it perfectly clear that he was all in favor of the makeover. Anne had given him three great kids and sacrificed a lot (including her body) to give them a good start in life. Joe told her he felt she deserved to have her body restored. Yes, they agreed, there were some "safety of surgery" worries. But they would do all the research together, find the right doctor, put some plans in place, and go for it!

And that's when I met them. We worked through all the possibilities, the questions, and the logistics. She had finished breast-feeding their youngest son a few months before, so she embarked on a program of exercise and weight loss to get down to her most realistic weight. And together she and her husband came to the conclusion that there is no perfect time—so we scheduled it.

Anne was able to take some time off from work, and her husband willingly signed up to take over the household duties for a few weeks (with the help of take-out food and a cleaning service). During that time, she told Joe, he would have to be nurse, pharmacy, and Mr. Mom—no small order!

The Mommy Makeover surgery went very smoothly. For the first few days, she was in a bit of pain, the kids were a little off balance and challenging, and her thoughts and emotions went through the roller coaster we had anticipated preoperatively. Were her new breasts too big—or not big enough? Is the swelling normal? (It was.) Had they wasted their money on this? Was she worth it?

Each day, though, brought improvement both physically and emotionally. The kids and dad settled into a new (clearly temporary) routine, and within a couple of weeks mom was back up and running through most of her usual activities. The house was still standing. The kids had actually had a few baths in the meantime. The boys even seemed to delight in *some* of dad's cooking. Her husband saw her as a whole new woman, not just physically but emotionally and energetically. He appreciated even more all she did every day to keep things going. He found her more attractive than ever, and it gave a nice spark to their relationship.

She took the kids to the neighborhood pool and found that because she was no longer worrying about how she looked, she was able to get into the pool and *play* with the kids. She was more willing, even excited, to get dressed up and go out with her husband or her girlfriends and have a good time. She was simply having more fun.

When she headed back to work, she took with her a new confidence—and a big smile. She no longer worried about looking older than her peers. She had a whole new focus on her job. And she found the courage to finally ask her boss for that overdue promotion … and he agreed.

The kids told me on one visit to my office, "Mom's just nicer." And "She smiles all the time." Her husband just beamed. "When Mom's happy, everybody's happy!"

This was a beautiful (and especially rewarding to me) example of how the Mommy Makeover can affect and improve the lives of a whole family.

I hope this book has given you some insight into some of the struggles a mom deals with in deciding to restore her body after childbirth. I hope I have shown you that, while there are some challenges to overcome, with planning (mentally, emotionally, and logistically), the Mommy Makeover can be a life-changing event for Mom and family alike.

If you are ready to take the next step on your journey to restoration, I encourage you to contact a board-certified plastic surgeon. You are always welcome to come visit me in Music City (Nashville). You can contact me via my website www.musiccityplasticsurgery. com or call my office at (615) 567-5716.

Printed in the USA
CPSIA information can be obtained
at www.ICGtesting.com
JSHW011417160824
R13664500003B/R136645PG68134JSX00039B/21